spinning

BY THE SAME AUTHOR:

The Power to Perform
The Performance Log
Precision Training

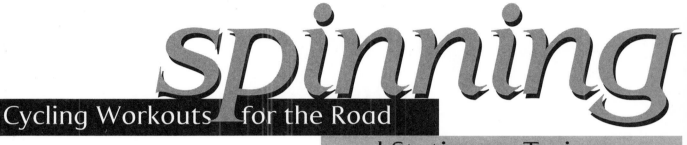

spinning

Cycling Workouts for the Road and Stationary Trainers

*For cycling, triathlon, duathlon, multisport,
mountainbiking, general fitness and fat loss*

Jon Ackland

REED

This book is dedicated to Kerri,
who always brings out the best in me.

Published by Reed Books, a division of Reed Publishing (NZ) Ltd,
39 Rawene Road, Birkenhead, Auckland 10.
Associated companies, branches and representatives throughout the world.

© Jon Ackland 1998
The author asserts his moral rights in the work.

ISBN 0 7900 0628 6

First published 1998
Printed in New Zealand

Acknowledgments

Thanks to the team at Performance Lab — Caroline Rutherford and Brendon Downey — who keep my life on an even keel and help me to cope with each magnificent day. Extra thanks also to Brendon for helping me develop some of the workouts in this book. Thanks to Craig Paterson for suggesting the idea for the book and for providing his book, *Advanced Turbo Training*, as a guide; to Jack Broome, Darren McKenzie Potter, Ric Reid, Theo Chapple, Dave Benson and Kelly Jackson for their ideas; to Russel and Denise Maylin, and to Peter Janssen and Peter Dowling of Reed Publishing.

Special thanks to Kent Butters of Litespeed, Cameron Brown, Rosie O'Neill and Tony Smith of Shephard Industries.

The equipment represented in this book is by:

  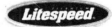

About the author

Jon Ackland is an exercise physiologist who has been working in the sports performance and training field for the last 15 years. As an 'applied sports scientist', he provides athletes and coaches with the training advice, testing and performance feedback needed to set up and refine high performance training systems.

Jon is the director of Performance Lab International, a company that helps athletes and coaches all over the world to improve performance. The company's goal is to provide 'cutting edge', quality information and training plans for all levels presented in a practical, commonsense format. In the four years that Performance Lab has been operational, its success in working with athletes and coaches has included two world records, eight national records, two world championships, numerous national titles, top Olympic performances, and many top ten placings in the world.

Jon holds a degree in science and a diploma of exercise science. Prior to setting up Performance Lab, he worked for the New Zealand Institute of Sport; under Jim Blair's supervision, with teams involved in New Zealand Rugby, Olympic yachting, America's Cup, Whitbread Around the World Yacht Race, New Zealand Basketball, New Zealand Hockey and New Zealand Skiing; and with many other top athletes of numerous sporting codes. His personal sporting background includes competitive school athletics, one national and three North Island rowing titles, five Ironmans and two representations at the World Ironman Triathlon championships in Hawaii.

Contents

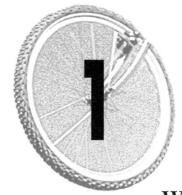

Getting started

Why spinning?

Most cycling-orientated athletes, and many people who simply wish to lose weight or get fit, have a stationary trainer. Having a stationary trainer at home means you don't have to train in the dark, the driving rain, the mayhem of 'road rage'-laden traffic or in the bone-numbing cold. Some people prefer not to travel to the gym simply to ride a stationary bike when they can do it in the comfort of their own home.

Despite the obvious advantages of using a stationary trainer, it is important to make sure you use them effectively. Many's the time I've been told by athletes that they didn't do the previous day's workout because the weather was rainy and terrible, but instead they got on their stationary trainer and, rather than doing their programmed 40-km hilly workout, they did 30 minutes of speedwork. The problem with this is that it changes the *balance* of their training. These athletes didn't have any way of converting their road training to their stationary trainer, and subsequently ended up not training as effectively.

The aim is smart, high-quality training that the body absorbs, not just doing indiscriminate garbage mileage. This requires a plan based on knowledge of what you want to achieve and how to go about it.

What we discovered was that there wasn't any information out there to help an athlete to fit a workout on a stationary trainer into a sports programme. Nor was there information for those wishing to improve their fitness or reduce body fat on a stationary bicycle. Sure, there are stationary trainer books out there that have the 'Butt Blaster' and 'Spin to Win' workouts, but they don't tell you where these workouts fit into a training build-up. There also seemed to be a lack of information for cyclists and athletes in sports that involve cycling on what to do in their workouts 'on the road'.

So this book is about maximising the quality of your cycle training, and your training in general — getting more performance for the same or less effort. Some of the material also appears in *Precision Training*, as a clear understanding of certain basic issues is essential in all forms of training. With additional information and training programmes that relate specifically to cycling and stationary trainers, *Spinning* will help you make more effective use of your stationary trainer, and improve your 'on the road' training.

This book is not only about using stationary trainers (windtrainers, turbo trainers) but also about integrating their use in combination with heart rate monitors to achieve effective, high-performance workouts.

Before we start, then, let's introduce the leading players.

And remember as you work through *Spinning*: the aim is not to make life hard for yourself. Have fun, train hard, live long and perspire!

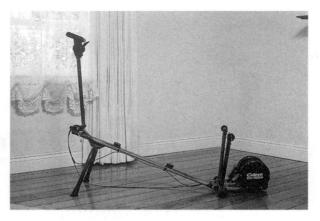

A stationary trainer

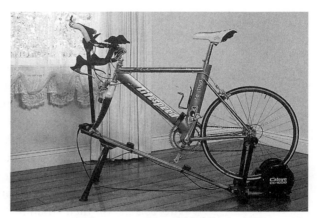

Stationary trainer with bike: ready to spin

The stationary trainer

Basically a stationary trainer is a supporting framework on which a cyclist can set their bike so that they can train inside, simulating their training on the road. Stationary trainers come in many different shapes and sizes, from types that hold the whole bike (back wheel locked in, with front forks attached) to trainers that support the back wheel only, to rollers (no support on two rolling cylinders — ride like hell and have great balance). Some can even be hooked up to a video game format where you see yourself as a computer-generated rider.

Then of course there are complete stationary cycles, of the type commonly used in gyms, and exercycles as well.

Why use a trainer?

- To avoid the rain.
- Safety — it can be dangerous to train on the road at night.
- Easier to concentrate on technique.
- Can be more time efficient.
- Can get more than one thing done at once (e.g. train and read over notes).
- To avoid the traffic.

Stationary trainers are almost a necessity in winter for athletes who work 9–5, as it is very difficult to find daylight training time during the week.

The heart

The heart is a muscle located under the rib cage (nearly in the centre of the chest), that pumps blood around the body. Why would it want to do this? Because your blood contains oxygen and oxygen is the fuel that makes the muscles work. Without oxygen the muscles would fail to operate and would die — so would you, for that matter. The blood also transports, delivers and removes other substances.

So if your muscles need oxygen, even at rest, they require blood; if they require more blood, it needs to be pumped by the heart. The harder an athlete works the more fuel, or oxygen, they require, and the more blood must be sent around the body — the result is a higher heart rate. That's why resting heart rates are low and exercising heart rates are high. The heart rate is the body's 'rev counter', measuring how much work the body is doing.

The complete sequence of a single heart beat follows a specific rhythm over and over again. This rhythm is actually a sequence of electrical impulses in the heart that occur in a pattern. This pattern forms a continuous repetitive electrical wave.

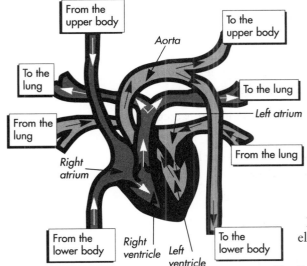

Fig. 1.1: The heart

The monitor

ECGs (electrocardiographs) have long been in use in hospitals. 'Electro' simply means electric, while 'cardio' means heart, and 'graph', surprisingly enough, means graph. So an ECG graphs the electricity generated by the heart in a wave. The wave is repeated over and over with each beat of the heart in a rhythmical sequence. This is used in hospitals to see if the patient's heart is operating correctly. If the rhythmical sequence changes, the heart is not beating correctly.

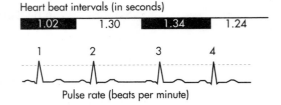

Fig. 1.2: The ECG — graphing the electrical activity of the heart

If you can measure the wave, you can measure the heart rate, which is taken as the main 'electrical pulse' of the heart occurs in each beat. And this is where the heart rate monitor comes in. Originally conceived as a measure of effort and fitness, portable wireless heart rate monitors were produced by Dr Seppo Saynajakangas in the early 1980s to help athletes to train more effectively.

The chest strap on the heart rate monitor has two electrodes that pick up the electrical pulse from the athlete's heart, and this is transmitted wirelessly to the wrist watch, or receiver. The wrist watch displays the pulse, or heart rate, providing extra information to the athlete on the body's physiological response to the exercise. Heart rate monitors have had an enormous impact on training and sport and have brought technology and sports/training science to athletes at all levels.

So why use a heart rate monitor?

- It acts as a 'rev counter' to give a precise measure or index of exercise intensity. You can actually measure how hard you are working.

- It allows you to individualise your programme so that you exercise at your pace, not someone else's.

- Your progress can be measured. As you become fitter, your heart rate at any given speed drops. Resting heart rate also drops.

- Because you witness improvement it's very motivational.

- Because your training suits you, it is of higher quality — that means less wasted training.

- It gives you an objective view of how hard you are working.

- It is a good indicator of fatigue (heart rate elevated in the morning) and other training variables.

- Because you know how hard you are working, you make fewer training errors and are less likely to suffer from overtraining and injury.
- You can be more specific about your training.

There are two parts to a heart rate monitor — the receiver (the wrist bit), and the transmitter and strap (the chest bit).

The strap that is worn around the chest has two electrodes which pick up the pulse rate. This is transmitted to the wrist watch (no wires!) by the transmitter on the strap (magic!). The receiver displays the heart rate.

The heart rate monitor can:

- display heart rate.
- set target training zones (it beeps if your heart rate is above or below the training zone).
- record average training heart rate for the training session.
- record heart rate at intervals.
- record heart rate for the full duration of the workout.
- also contain time, alarm, and stopwatch functions.

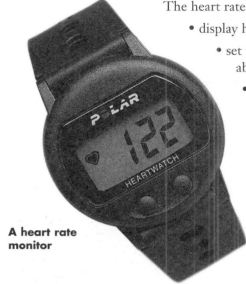

A heart rate monitor

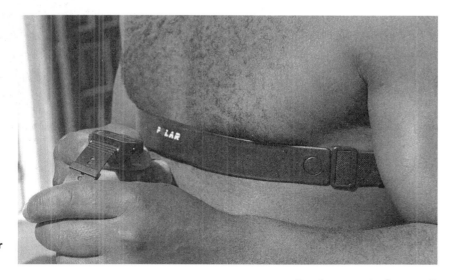

Heart rate monitor and chest strap

The combination

Combining the use of heart rate monitors and stationary trainers allows you to develop very specific schedules that maximise performance for the time you put in. This is the essence of quality training.

Of course, there are both good points and bad points about using stationary trainers.

The downside

- It's hot.
- It's boring.
- It's tiring.
- It's uncomfortable.

However, these negatives can all be overcome quite simply, as we shall see a little further on in the book.

The upside

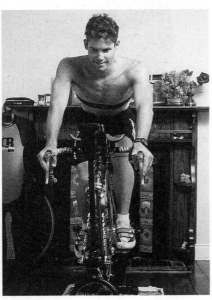

- Very effective workouts.
- Excellent control of your training.
- It doesn't rain, snow or blow a howling gale indoors.
- You don't get as many punctures.
- It's safer indoors.
- You are closer to home if you get tired or the phone rings.

The bottom line

Stationary trainer workouts make a good supplement to your 'on the road' training.

Stationary trainer workout using a heart rate monitor

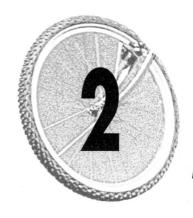

Plan your training — periodisation

We've discussed the basics, now let's go through a brief overview of how you plan your training.

We'll start with seasons, then break the seasons into periods and the periods into subphases, and finally end up with a training programme where you completely understand the three major questions in a training programme:

1. How far/long do you go?

2. What do you do when you get out there?

3. How hard do you go?

Off-season

This is the transition or active recovery phase. It usually lasts between 2–12 weeks, although it can last for as long as 10 months.

Training during this phase should be fun! Recreational training will rest the body and mind while retaining performance potential for the build-up that follows. The off-season is essentially a balancing act between recovery and maintaining fitness. The best way to achieve this is to do 'fun' workouts, or incorporate training into things you like to do (e.g. cycle to a café). You can also do 'like' sport training — for example, mountainbiking is very good for maintaining your road cycling form.

The key is to recover mentally. Most cyclists can recover physically in a very short space of time, but to recover mentally — to be enthusiastic to train 'full on' again — takes a little longer. You need to remove everything that reminds you of training. Don't train in the same way, on the same courses, at the same times — do something different!

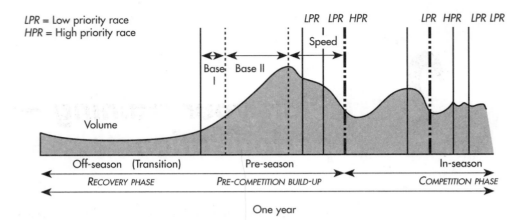

LPR = Low priority race
HPR = High priority race

LPR LPR HPR   LPR HPR LPR LPR

Speed

Base   Base II
  I

Volume

Off-season (Transition)   Pre-season   In-season

RECOVERY PHASE   PRE-COMPETITION BUILD-UP   COMPETITION PHASE

One year

Characteristics
- Recovery (physical and mental).
- 'Like' sport training.
- Light low-intensity maintenance training.

- Slow progressive build-up in training from off-season to competition levels.
- Base training is predominantly low-intensity continuous training.
- Speed training carries an element of base training but also includes speedwork (intervals, sprints, time trials and races).

- Maintenance of race readiness.
- Manipulation of base and speed training.
- Rotating of training to peak for high priority races, recover and then build up again.
- Low priority races (LPR) — warm-ups or races that you 'train through' in preparation for peak, high priority races.

Fig 2.1: Training seasons

Pre-season

This is the preparatory phase, or build-up, and it usually lasts between 10–20 weeks. It is the time to prepare and train, to build up from the off-season to high performance for your major competition(s). Pre-season is broken into two major training periods: Base and Speed.

In-season

This is the competition or racing phase. It can last between 1–6 months; the norm is 8–12 weeks. In-season may consist of a single peak for a specific goal event or several peaks that require peaking, dropping form, and peaking again.

Many cyclists think they can peak for a whole competing season. This is, unfortunately, impossible, so training must be based around up to six goal events per year. For example, 1–4 short races (e.g. standard course triathlon, road races, mountain bike races) are tolerable for most athletes. For long distance races (e.g. Ironman, Coast to Coast, tours) the number of races drops to 1–2. You may still do many more low-priority races, but they are not races you aim to peak in.

Pre-season in detail — training periods

As we've seen, pre-season is divided into two training periods, Base and Speed. Base is the mileage phase and Speed is competition-specific conditioning.

Base aims to build 'fitness', recovery and tolerance to training, to allow the athlete/player to do effective speedwork (the 'go fast' part). This results in a maximum potential performance. It is also used to show the athlete the distance or duration of the competition. If you look closely at training, Base is further broken down into endurance and strength endurance while Speed is, as it states, speed.

Fig 2.2: Training periods

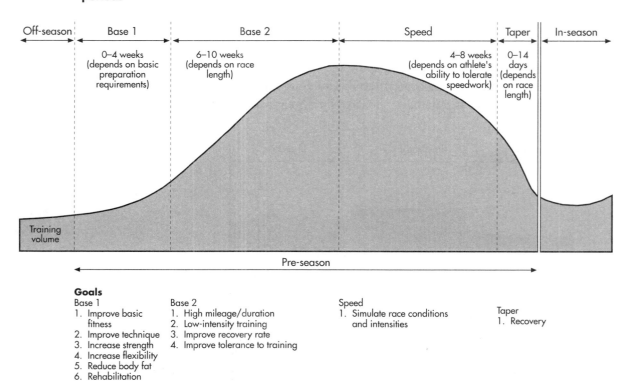

| Off-season | Base 1 | Base 2 | Speed | Taper | In-season |

- Base 1: 0–4 weeks (depends on basic preparation requirements)
- Base 2: 6–10 weeks (depends on race length)
- Speed: 4–8 weeks (depends on athlete's ability to tolerate speedwork)
- Taper: 0–14 days (depends on race length)

Training volume

Pre-season

Goals

Base 1
1. Improve basic fitness
2. Improve technique
3. Increase strength
4. Increase flexibility
5. Reduce body fat
6. Rehabilitation

Base 2
1. High mileage/duration
2. Low-intensity training
3. Improve recovery rate
4. Improve tolerance to training

Speed
1. Simulate race conditions and intensities

Taper
1. Recovery

Base

TECHNIQUE/ENDURANCE (BASE 1)

Endurance is designed to get the athlete conditioned to training. It takes account of initial fitness and allows time to address weaker factors in the training. Once endurance training has been carried out the cyclist will be 'fit' enough to cope with further, more strenuous types of training. Endurance enables the athlete to complete the race distance, or begin to, for longer races. Establishing good technique is vital during this phase; the emphasis is on volume and technique.

STRENGTH ENDURANCE (BASE 2)

Strength endurance can now be trained. If endurance allows you to complete the race, strength endurance gives you the ability to apply more 'grunt' (strength, power, force). An example of this in cycling could be that endurance training is pedalling easily up to or above race distance; strength endurance is riding the same distance in a big gear (low cadence — uphill and flat).

Strength endurance moves from slowly increasing the muscular effort of the activity to maintaining the muscular effort and applying speed.

Speed

Speed is the time to simulate competition conditions and intensities. The athlete's body responds by adapting to this training, and their performance therefore goes up. If training is showing your body what will happen on

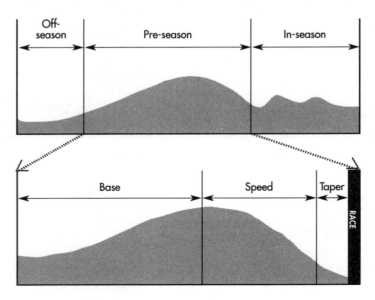

Fig 2.3: Pre-season — Base and Speed phases

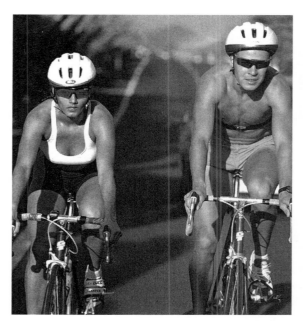

Periodisation can work for an individual or equally for training partners.

race day so that it can adapt to it, speed makes this more and more specific to the race as it draws nearer.

Speed generally moves from longer, slower training to shorter, faster training — from tempo training to anaerobic threshold/ maximum steady-state pace to long sprints, short sprints, power and overspeed, in that order.

Taper

The taper is actually part of the Speed phase as speedwork is still performed during the taper. A taper is a gradual reduction in training volume to allow the athlete to recover fully before the race, so that they are capable of maximum performance on race day. Too long a taper and the cyclist's form begins to drop, too short a taper and recovery is incomplete and they will compete tired.

A taper is a very personal part of training, as what suits one competitor will not suit another. Tapers generally last between 2–14 days, depending on the competition. The longer the duration of the event, the longer the taper.

Training subphases

Technique, endurance, strength endurance and speed
We've looked at seasons and periods, now we look at what we do in the Base and Speed periods.

Subphases: types of training
Intensity and volume are combined to give different types of training! Here is how the types of training progress through the programme to peak.

The first thing you need to be able to do is *perform the action* properly. That's what correct *technique* is all about. Then you need to *perform the action properly for a long time*. That's *endurance*. You need to get 'fit' doing the technique.

Then you need to *perform the action properly for a long time with 'grunt'*. There's no point in being technically good and fit if you can't apply the

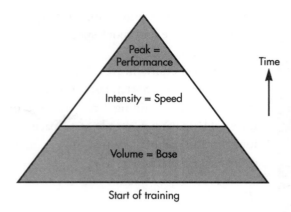

Fig 2.4: Progression
of training from Base
(volume) to Speed
(intensity) to peak.

power. That's *strength/strength endurance*. Finally, you add pace — you need *to perform the action properly for a long time with 'grunt' and pace*. This is speed. In other words, development occurs through the progression from technique to endurance to strength/strength endurance to speed (see fig 2.5).

This is how performance is developed. Intensity and volume must be combined sequentially into types of training to improve performance.

Training history also affects performance and peak. The longer you have been doing the sport, the more you can cope with. The more you can cope with, the more speedwork you can do. And the more speedwork you can do, the faster you will go in competition.

Training history affects how much technique you can do, which affects how much endurance you can do, which affects how much strength/ strength endurance you can do, which affects how much speed you can do, which determines how high you can peak.

Subphases

So, Base and Speed can be further broken down into subphases. These are small 'chunks' of training (usually around 3–4 weeks long) where specific forms of training are emphasised. These may be aspects of technique, endurance, strength endurance or speed.

The table on page 14 represents a breakdown of the pre-season into Base and Speed periods, and then into subphases. Note that there is a logical progression from the preparation phase, through to sport-specific strength endurance training, and finally to speed training. Training also moves from less competition-specific to more competition-specific.

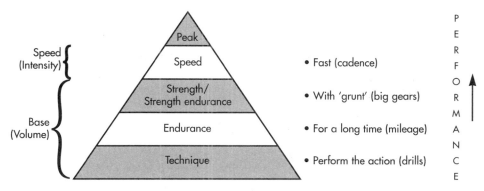

Fig 2.5: Full progression of training showing the types of training in Base that progress through to other types of training during speedwork to peak.

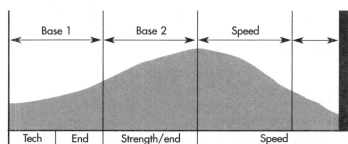

Fig 2.6: The progression from technique to endurance to strength endurance to speed within a training programme.

The following pages provide a more detailed explanation of subphases 1–9 so that you can apply these easily to your daily workouts.

Base phase

1. Preparation (easy)

EASY TRAINING/GETTING FIT

This involves easy conditioning, starting back into a more structured training programme from your off-season and getting your body ready for the training ahead. All problems (muscle and strength imbalances, injuries and rehabilitation) are dealt with before the training load increases. This phase can be avoided if you are already well conditioned, or could take many weeks if problems need to be resolved. Technique should be concentrated on. You need to work on performing the action. Easy training occurs early in Base, once to twice a week. This subphase usually lasts 0–4 weeks.

SPECIFICS: Light/easy conditioning (aerobic)

EFFORT: Easy conversation pace (50–60% effort)
Low muscular effort

TRAINING HEART RATES: Long slow distance (60–75% HR^{max})

SUBPHASES	PERIODS		SEASON
1. Preparation (easy)	Base 1 Endurance (conditioning)	} BASE PHASE	P R E S E A S O N
2. Load 3. High load 4. Load/speed	Base 2 Strength/endurance		
5. Low-speed work 6. High-speed work 7. Sprints 8. Power 9. Overspeed	Speed (if needed) (if needed) (if needed)	} SPEED PHASE	

2. Load

GETTING STRONGER

Load is the beginning of strength endurance. At this point the cyclist is fit and conditioned enough to start to increase the training effort without fear of injury and to get the most out of it. Hill training is used to build strength endurance, from more moderate shorter climbs to longer, steeper multiple climbs. You have, through your training, reached a point where you have shown your body how to perform the action for a long time with a moderate degree of grunt!

Load is emphasised in early Base, and would occur progressively from once to twice per week. This phase could last from 2–8 weeks (generally 4).

SPECIFICS: Strength endurance training

EFFORT: Easy conversation pace (60–70% effort; effort will obviously be slightly higher under load — 70–80%, no higher)
Medium muscular effort

TRAINING HEART RATES: During — N/A
Between — 60–75% HR^{max}

3. High load

GETTING STRONGER

This is an extension of strength endurance training. As the athlete becomes conditioned to load training, the load and the resistance is increased.

Cyclists may move from hill training to riding hills in a big gear. Big-gear hill training involves training on hills in gears 1–5 cogs (approximately based on conditioning/training history) higher than normal. Pedal cadence is low (30–50 rpm) and the aim is not to work too hard but to turn over a large gear so that the focus is on the legs not the lungs. Move from 1 to 3 or 4 cogs higher than the goal you would normally use on the hill. Use normal gears between hills to recover. 'Pure strength' training may also be applied to improve acceleration for cycle racing. This involves starting at the bottom of the hill in the biggest gear you have from an almost stationary speed. You then cycle only 15–30 pedal strokes up a hill until you almost stall, then turn and roll back down the hill.

Be very careful when doing this training as it is easy to become injured. Knees are particularly at risk. You should warm up at the start of your ride. Do a further warm-up on some hills before progressing to big-gear training. In cold conditions keep your knees warm and don't continue if your knees are at all irritated. Younger cyclists should skip this subphase.

Also be careful that this form of training does not affect your form as technique can deteriorate if you don't remain vigilant.

This further 'strengthens' the athlete and prepares them for the upcoming speedwork (in the subsequent subphase). You have, through your training, reached a point where you have shown your body how to perform the action for a long time, with grunt!

This phase is emphasised in the middle of Base. It should be applied from not at all to once or twice a week over a 2- to 8-week period (generally 4 weeks). Cyclists aged under 16 should avoid this phase.

SPECIFICS:	High strength endurance
EFFORT:	Easy conversation pace (60–75% effort; during high load 75–85% effort) High muscular effort
TRAINING HEART RATE:	During — N/A Between — LSD (60–75% HR^{max})

4. Load/speed

APPLYING STRENGTH (GRUNT, POWER) TO SPEED

Load/speed is the transition form of training that ties strength endurance training to speed training. It's often called conversion or transfer training. You can't just go immediately from high load, low speed to high speed, so load/speed is used to begin speed but maintain an aspect of strength. This allows a gradual progression to speed (your body hates anything sudden) and allows the strength to be applied to speed.

This form of training is similar to hills, in that you are deliberately overgeared for the situation. You introduce your body to your 'most used' race gear to improve your strength endurance. The cadence is dropped (40–60 rpm) so that your legs can get used to the gear without bringing the cardiovascular effort at the same time — this is saved for speedwork. Long intervals of 10–20 minutes can be used. Top cyclists can do up to 100–110 km of this form of training in a week, but young cyclists should avoid it.

A variation is to oscillate the cadence between 40 and 80 rpm. This begins to transfer the strength endurance gained at low cadences to speed by using slightly higher cadences. For example:

CADENCE (RPM)	TIME SPENT AT CADENCE	GEAR
80	1 min	52 × 16
70	2 min	52 × 16
60	3 min	52 × 16
50	3 min	52 × 16
40	3 min	52 × 16

You have, through your training, reached a point where you have shown your body how to perform the action, for a long time, with grunt and the beginnings of going fast.

This would occur from not at all to once or twice a week over a 2- to 8-week period (usually 2–4 weeks). This is emphasised at the end of Base. Cyclists aged under 16 should avoid this phase.

SPECIFICS: Strength endurance moving to speed endurance

EFFORT: Easy conversation pace (60–75% effort)
Medium muscular effort

TRAINING HEART RATE: During — N/A
Between — LSD (60–75% HR^{max})

Speed phase

You are now ready for the Speed phase. You have conditioned your body, dealt with any problems and improved your strength, so you can begin to increase the tempo of your training. This is when the real work starts.

The following subphases are progressively combined into between 1–3 speed sessions per week (1 = novice, 3 = elite) over the last 4–8 weeks of the Speed phase. Racing and competition is often a better form of speed training (more specific) and can be substituted for a speed session.

Speedwork is very intense and demanding. Too much speedwork can quickly overfatigue a cyclist and destroy a build-up. As a rule of thumb, 10 percent of your training in your biggest speedwork week can be at high speed work (6–9) or higher, or 20 percent low speed work (5–8) or higher; 80 percent easy (1), load (2), high load (3) and load/speed (4). Each of the following phases is initiated progressively each week during the Speed phase.

5. Low-speed work

THE BEGINNINGS OF SPEED CONDITIONING

Up-tempo is the beginning of conditioning for speed. This form of training is faster than easy conversation pace but not as fast as 10- to 60-minute race pace. You should be training fast at about 70–75 percent effort, feeling comfortable, strong, in control and not 'hammering' (Ironman, tour race pace). Because this form of training is only moderately intense, the interval periods can be quite long (10–20 mins).

This would occur once or twice a week and would be gradually phased in over a period of 2–4 weeks (usually 2). The emphasis is at the end of Base for competitions under four hours and at the start of Speed for competitions over four hours.

You have, through your training, reached a point where you have shown your body how to perform the action for a long time with grunt, fast.

SPECIFICS:	Long intervals at tempo pace (Ironman race pace) should feel fast and strong
EFFORT:	Moderately difficult to converse (70–75% effort) Medium muscular effort
TRAINING HEART RATE:	During — UT (75–85% HR^{max}) Between — LSD (60–75% HR^{max})

6. High-speed work

GETTING FAST IN TERMS OF ENDURANCE (HIGH AEROBIC SPEED)

Anaerobic threshold: anaerobic threshold is defined as the highest intensity that an athlete can hold for approximately one hour. This equates to around 40-km time-trial pace on your bike.

Anaerobic threshold training can be conducted as time trials or as less psychologically demanding intervals (frequently between 4–10 minutes). This improves your anaerobic threshold pace. It also allows your race pace to come up, or improves high steady-state race pace.

This subphase lasts between 2–8 weeks (usually 1–4 weeks). It is emphasised at the start of Speed for competitions of less than 4 hours, and in the middle of Speed for competitions over four hours.

SPECIFICS: Short intervals (16-km run or 40-km bike time trial pace); you should feel like you are hammering (anaerobic threshold)

EFFORT: Difficult to converse (75–85% effort)
                      Medium muscular effort

TRAINING HEART RATE: During — AT (85–95% HR^{max})
                      Between — LSD (60–75% HR^{max})

7. *Sprints (extensive/intensive sprints) — long and short*
GETTING FAST IN TERMS OF LONG AND SHORT SPRINTING
(LOW AND HIGH ANAEROBIC SPEED)

Sprints improve your anaerobic speed — your ability to hold very high speeds for very short distances. Sprints break down into two parts.

EXTENSIVE SPRINTS: long sprints (between 45 seconds and 4 minutes is typical) are used to improve the ability to sustain sprint speed at the start or end of a race, to bridge gaps, to break away from the peloton close to the finish or to initiate breakaways.

INTENSIVE SPRINTS: short sprints (usually between 10 seconds and 1 minute) are used to improve ability at top sprinting speed. Intensive sprints can be broken into uphill (50 m), crest (30 m uphill/30 m over the top) and on the flat (200–400 m). Uphill sprints occur during the load and high-load phase, crest occurs in the load/speed phase, and flat occurs in speed.

These types of training occur once or twice a week over a 1–4-week period (usually 2 weeks). This is emphasised in the middle to end of Speed.

SPECIFICS: Extensive sprints (long sprints) are 2–4-min sprints.
                      Intensive sprints (short sprints) are 10 sec to 1 min 30 sec sprints (anaerobic lactic and alactic)

EFFORT: Very difficult to converse (90–100% effort)
                      High muscular effort

TRAINING HEART RATE: During — N/A (above 95% HR^{max})
                      Between — LSD (60–75% HR^{max})

8. Power (acceleration)

GETTING FAST IN TERMS OF EXPLOSIVE SPEED
(VERY HIGH ANAEROBIC SPEED)

Power training improves explosive ability. Power training is used to improve the ability in cycling to attack a rider or the peloton in an initial 'jump'. Power training can be conducted using plyometrics or big gear wind-outs, or by using a dip in the road to gain speed down a hill in a big gear, then sprinting using the same gear up a short climb on the other side of the dip and stopping when you are not 'on top of the gear'. You should feel strong (i.e. you should not labour to turn the gear over).

This subphase can occur once or twice a week over a 1–4-week period. The subphase is emphasised towards the end of Speed.

SPECIFICS:	Explosive acceleration (anaerobic alactic)
EFFORT:	100% effort High muscular effort
TRAINING HEART RATE:	During — N/A Between — (60–75% HR^{max})

9. Overspeed

GETTING YOU FAST IN TERMS OF SPEED OF MOVEMENT
(TOP-END BIOMECHANICS SPEED — OVER PACE MOVEMENT OF LIMBS)

Overspeed training involves increasing muscular contraction speed, which is the final aspect of speedwork. Downhill spinning sprints in cycling (sprinting downhill in a small gear at a high cadence) and motor pacing (high-cadence training drafting behind a vehicle to decrease the effects of wind resistance) are useful forms of overspeed.

SPECIFICS:	Short downhill sprint intervals or motor pacing (drafting behind a motor vehicle) at above race pace speed to enhance muscle contraction speed
EFFORT:	Moderate/low load and high speed Low muscular effort
TRAINING HEART RATE:	During — N/A Between — (60–75% HR^{max})

In most cases, once you start to use a training intensity you don't stop. It may be slowly initiated and progressively increased between 1–3 weeks before you focus on a specific training subphase, and will reach its peak emphasis and then be maintained as other training phases are initiated.

Putting the subphases together

So there it is: those are all the ingredients. But training is like cooking — it's not the ingredients that count, it's how they are put together.

To put the ingredients together successfully you first need an experienced athlete or coach to advise you. They can use their experience to take the guesswork out of your training and will save you having to learn the hard way. Be specific about what you require in training for your event. You may not use every subphase as you may not have enough time, or may not require some of the intensities (e.g. sprint training will not greatly improve your time-trial ability), or you may want to spend more time on a specific phase that is your weakness.

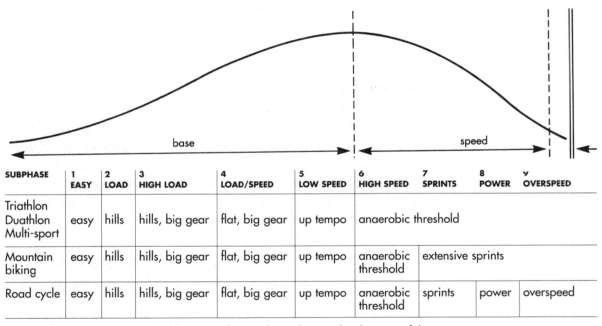

SUBPHASE	1 EASY	2 LOAD	3 HIGH LOAD	4 LOAD/SPEED	5 LOW SPEED	6 HIGH SPEED	7 SPRINTS	8 POWER	9 OVERSPEED
Triathlon Duathlon Multi-sport	easy	hills	hills, big gear	flat, big gear	up tempo	anaerobic threshold			
Mountain biking	easy	hills	hills, big gear	flat, big gear	up tempo	anaerobic threshold	extensive sprints		
Road cycle	easy	hills	hills, big gear	flat, big gear	up tempo	anaerobic threshold	sprints	power	overspeed

NOTE: Subphases timing in a build-up can change depending on the duration of the race. (See *Precision Training* or *The Power to Perform*.)

Fig 2.7: Subphase requirements for cycling in various sports

3 Training intensities

There are three major parts to training:

- Volume: the amount of training (measured in time or distance).
- Intensity: the energy or effort required for a specific form of training (measured objectively by heart rate, or subjectively by perceived effort).
- Performance: level of ability (measured in outcome, time, distance or placing).

Generally, volume comes before intensity. Changes in volume and intensity (and types of training) change performance.

VOLUME + INTENSITY = PERFORMANCE

In most training programmes, volume moves progressively up, then down, as intensity builds. Intensity generally moves progressively up.

Let's take a closer look at the intensity part of training.

The energy systems

First we need to know a little about how the body works. The body uses two main energy systems, one of which breaks down into two further parts. These systems are:

1. The ANAEROBIC energy system, which breaks down into the alactic (immediate) and lactic (non-oxidative) subsystems;

2. The AEROBIC energy system (oxidative).

The ANAEROBIC system is used during high-intensity exercise where energy demands exceed aerobic metabolism. In other words, this system is used when you are exercising without your muscles using oxygen; in sprinting, for example.

21

The ANAEROBIC ALACTIC system is used during very high-intensity exercise (maximum effort under 10–20 seconds) and supplies immediate energy. It does not require oxygen to function (anaerobic) and no lactic acid is produced (alactic).

The ANAEROBIC LACTIC system 'kicks in' just before the anaerobic alactic system runs out, and does not require oxygen to function (anaerobic). It does, however, produce lactic acid as a major by-product of energy production (lactic). The anaerobic lactic system is used in moderately intense activity lasting from 10 seconds to 2–3 minutes. It is used when oxygen is in short supply or when there is a complete lack of oxygen.

The aerobic energy system takes in, transports and uses oxygen. It requires the presence of oxygen to function. It comes into play after about 2 minutes of intense exercise and is the main source of energy after 3–4 minutes.

The aerobic energy system is used for moderately intensive exercise and is developed and maintained through cardiovascular exercise, such as cycling, running, swimming, kayaking and rowing. Cardiovascular exercise stimulates the cardiovascular system (heart and blood vessels) and is any exercise that increases heart rate. It is also called cardiorespiratory exercise because it improves the ability of the heart and lungs to deliver oxygen to the working muscles. Why do you need to know this? Because your training intensities are built around them!

The aerobic system can be tested by assessing VO_{2max}; a basic test is given in Appendix 3. For a full explanation see *The Power to Perform*.

Training intensities and heart rate

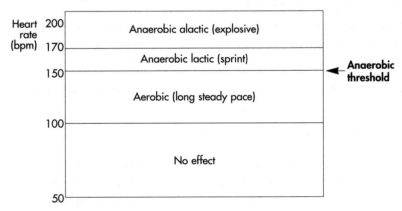

Fig 3.1: Anaerobic and aerobic zones in relation to heart rate

Understanding the 'hardness' or intensity of your training is the key to understanding how a progressive, balanced training programme is put together. While novice and élite athletes may be poles apart when it comes to how fast they train and race, the intensity (not speed) of the work each group does in each phase of their training is the same.

Training intensities have traditionally been categorised in many different ways, but they can easily be broken down into three basic types. Starting with the lowest intensity and moving up to the highest, these intensities are:

1. Low intensity: easy–medium;

2. Submaximal intensity: medium–hard;

3. High intensity: hard–very hard.

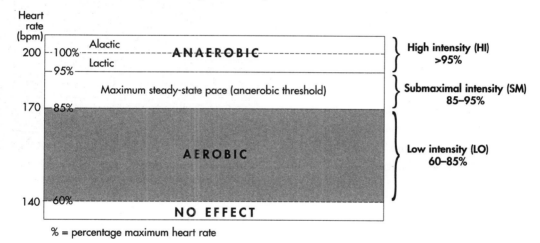

Fig 3.2: Training intensities

Low-intensity (LO) training is aerobic exercise (with oxygen) which can be performed for long periods of time. High-intensity (HI) training is anaerobic (without oxygen). High-intensity exercise (basically sprinting) can only be performed for brief periods before complete temporary fatigue occurs and you have to rest.

Submaximal-intensity (SM) training occurs at what some regard as the threshold or crossover between LO and HI training. This is the maximum steady-state pace, or anaerobic threshold pace, you can hold (20 minutes– 1 hour).

Low-intensity (LO) training

Easy to Medium (60–85 percent Heart Rate Max)

LO training gives you basic aerobic fitness and muscular conditioning and it will improve your ability to metabolise (use) fat as an energy source. LO training, which can also be used to aid recovery, can be broken down into three types. These too have an order of intensity:

1. Active recovery (AR).

2. Long slow distance (LSD).

3. Up-tempo (UT).

Active recovery occurs at the easy end of the LO training range, while up-tempo occurs just below submaximal intensity (SM) training. LO training is performed at approximately 60–85 percent of your HR^{max}.

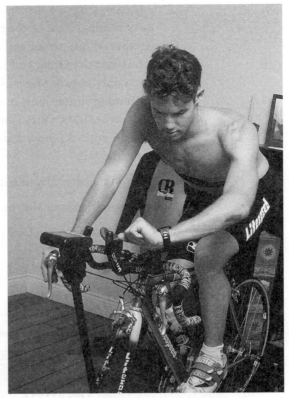

Constant monitoring of your training helps to ensure the correct intensity is maintained.

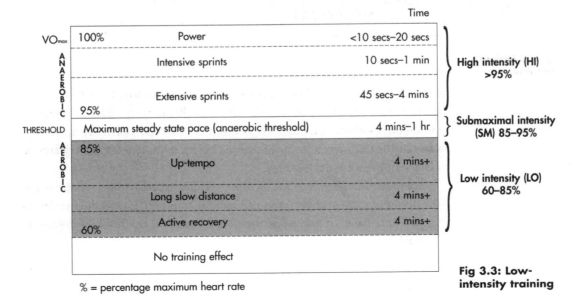

			Time		
VO_{max} 100%		Power	<10 secs–20 secs	⎫	
A N A E R O B I C		Intensive sprints	10 secs–1 min	⎬	**High intensity (HI)** >95%
		Extensive sprints	45 secs–4 mins	⎭	
95%					
THRESHOLD		Maximum steady state pace (anaerobic threshold)	4 mins–1 hr	⎬	**Submaximal intensity (SM) 85–95%**
A E R O B I C	85%	Up-tempo	4 mins+	⎫	
		Long slow distance	4 mins+	⎬	**Low intensity (LO) 60–85%**
	60%	Active recovery	4 mins+	⎭	
		No training effect			

% = percentage maximum heart rate

Fig 3.3: Low-intensity training

Most athletes will work at the middle to low end of this range (AR, LSD) most of the time until up-tempo training begins in preparation for speedwork.

If you do not have access to a heart rate monitor or you don't wish to use heart rates as a guide to training intensity, LO pace can be described as an easy to medium effort (if you can't comfortably hold a conversation at this pace, i.e. you're gasping, then you're going too fast!).

Active recovery (<60% HR^max)

Active recovery is performed at approximately 60 percent of HR^{max}, at the lowest end of the low-intensity training heart rate range. It is only used in training to assist recovery, for example by removing waste products from the muscles (warm down), or when you feel tired.

AR should be used on those days when you feel too tired to do your intended workout. But if after 10–15 minutes of training you still feel tired, go home and have a rest! Further training on that day will do more harm than good.

If you feel you need a day off altogether — take it (and forget about training until tomorrow).

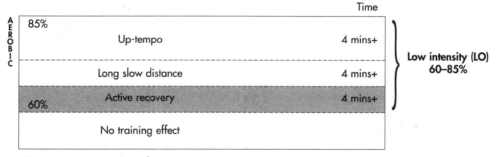

% = percentage maximum heart rate

Fig 3.4: Active recovery

Long slow distance (60–75% HR^MAX)

Long slow distance is performed at approximately 60–75 percent of HR^{max}. LSD is the most used training zone. Most of your training will be in this zone. It is often called the 'mileage zone' — the zone where you do most of your mileage, aerobic conditioning training.

This zone improves endurance, familiarises your body with training, improves efficiency, assists in weight control and improves strength or muscular endurance. This is not a very specific intensity, just an easy pace at which to hold a conversation. The pace will improve as you get fitter.

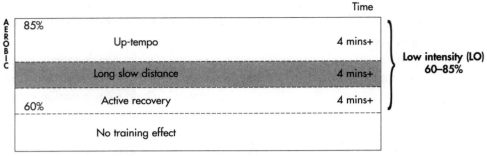

% = percentage maximum heart rate

Up-tempo training (75–85% HR^{max})

Up-tempo is performed at approximately 75–85 percent of HR^{max}, and is an intermediate intensity that bridges the gap between LO and higher intensity training. It's the start of aerobic (endurance) speed work. It conditions the body to the beginnings of 'going faster'.

Time

A E R O B I C	85%		
		Up-tempo	4 mins+
		Long slow distance	4 mins+
	60%	Active recovery	4 mins+
		No training effect	

Low intensity (LO)
60–85%

% = percentage maximum heart rate

The effects of low-intensity training

This intensity improves basic aerobic and muscular conditioning (including muscular endurance), speeds recovery and increases your tolerance to training. These training adaptations enable you to cope with the speedwork to come and condition you for the more intense, more specific work to come.

Low-intensity training also improves your ability to metabolise or use fat as a source of energy. This means you are better able to race over long distances with less likelihood of 'bonking'. That is valuable for endurance athletes and assists in fat loss.

Submaximal intensity (SM) training

Medium to Hard (85–95 percent Heart Rate Max)

SM training occurs at maximum steady-state/anaerobic threshold (approximately 85–95 percent of HR^{max}). It raises your maximum steady-state pace (often called 'anaerobic threshold pace') or race pace.

These days, 'anaerobic threshold' is a term frowned upon by sports scientists. This is because there is no absolute threshold but rather a 'grey area' where your body moves from functioning at a mainly aerobic level (where most of your energy needs are being met by oxygen) to functioning at a mainly anaerobic level (you can't take in enough oxygen to sustain your current level of exercise intensity). Therefore, the term 'submaximal intensity' is used to describe training that corresponds with that 'grey area' where you are exercising hard enough to border on going into oxygen debt, starting to puff heavily or starting to sprint. SM training is usually about 85–95 percent of HR^{max}, although these percentages vary a lot depending on your conditioning and the phase of training you are in.

In simple terms, SM training pace is medium to hard. You should find it difficult to converse at this pace.

The effects of submaximal intensity training

Various types of SM training will improve steady-state racing (time trial, average race pace) speed and muscle endurance.

Submaximal intensity training is the cornerstone of your racing speed.

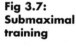

**Fig 3.7:
Submaximal
training**

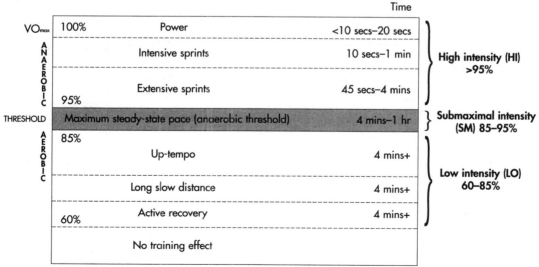

% = percentage maximum heart rate

High-intensity (HI) training

Hard to Very Hard (95–100 percent Heart Rate Max)

HI training is anaerobic, and performed at approximately 95–100 percent of HR^{max}. It bears some similarity to SM training, but it also improves your ability to cope with sprinting (acceleration, top speed and speed endurance), sprint recovery (oxygen debt), and high levels of exertion.

High-intensity training can be broken down into:

1. Sprinting (extensive) — ES.

2. Sprinting (intensive) — IS.

3. Power (acceleration) — PWR.

To exercise at above 95 percent of your HR^{max} means sprinting. It is the only time in training when you should let all the brakes off and go for it. To some extent, it is hard to define and monitor exact heart rate levels at this intensity. If you are using a heart rate monitor, it is assumed that heart rates must be above 95 percent HR^{max} to have the desired effect. But it is better to use the duration of the sprint to control intensity. Why? Because in very short sprints your heart rate will not reach a constant, meaningful level. HI training pace can be described as hard to very hard. You should not be able to talk. Actually, even thinking should be difficult!

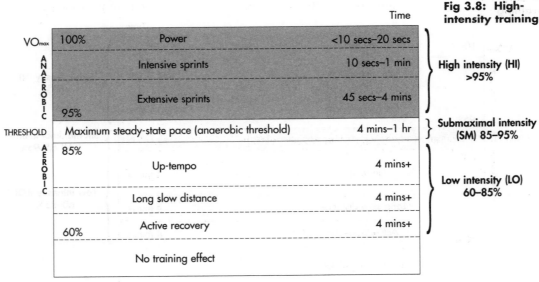

Fig 3.8: High-intensity training

% = percentage maximum heart rate

What makes up high-intensity (HI) training?

Extensive sprints (> 95% HR^max)

Extensive sprints involve a 90–95 percent effort, and last between 45 seconds and 4 minutes.

These are long sprints, which are used to condition your body to extended sprinting (speed endurance). They are used for cycle racing, any multisport races that involve some aspect of cycle racing in a bunch (peloton), for long breakaways and bridging the gap between bunches, and starts.

Intensive sprints

Intensive sprints are short, lasting between 10 seconds and 1 minute, but they involve 100 percent effort. They are used to improve your top sprinting speed and speed endurance. This intensity is mainly used in a top speed sport, as in sprinting for the line in a cycling race.

Power sprints

Power sprints involve 100 percent effort, and last no more than 10–20 seconds. They are used to develop explosive ability (efforts generally lasting less than 10 seconds) and acceleration. This improves your 'jump' of 'kick' in cycling.

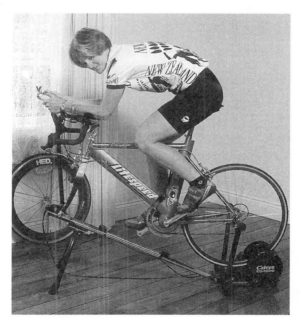

**Sprint practice
while spinning**

THE VALUE OF HIGH-INTENSITY TRAINING

High-intensity training improves your recovery from oxygen debt and your ability to sustain pace in oxygen debt (lactate tolerance). It is good for fast starts and finishes, as well as explosive acceleration and sprinting. In cycling it is very good for pushing up and over hills, breakaways, sprint 'primes', sprint finishes, and starts, and for bridging the gap between bunches.

Acceleration, top speed and speed endurance can be developed separately or in combination, generally progressing from ES to IS and finally to PW. Overspeed (an aspect of HI: lighter load and a muscle contraction slightly higher than race pace) can also be used in some sports. Overspeed is not an intensity as it is more to improve muscle contraction speed (biomechanical) than to improve cardiorespiratory function (physiological).

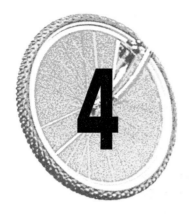

Calculating training heart rates

Calculating training intensities

Two ways to calculate your training intensities are presented here. The easiest but least accurate is to look them up in the tables. The second, more accurate method is by assessing your resting and maximum heart rates and doing an anaerobic threshold test. Assess which method you should use in the table below:

RECOMMENDATIONS/TYPE	METHOD
Novice/General Fitness	1
Beginner Sports	1
Semi-Competitive	1 or 2
Competitive	2
Elite	2

NOTE: If your heart rates don't feel right, you are probably different from the normal — use method 2.

Once you have worked out your training heart rates write them in the spaces provided at the end of this chapter and in the specific programme section of the book (pages 41–43). Either design your own programme using the instructions provided in *The Power to Perform*, or use the programmes provided in this book.

If you are using a programme from another source (from another book, magazine, coach or of your own design), you will need to read the subphases carefully and either incorporate the heart rates and training specifics, or translate the training terminology and adapt it for the programme.

Method 1: Assessing training intensities through tables — very easy method

(For novice recreational athletes and general fitness)

Look up your heart rates based on age and sex.

MALE

AGE	LD			SM	HI			*HR MAX
	AR (R)	LSD (AFL)	UT (HA)	AT (AT)	ES (RLZ)	IS	PWR	
15–20	<140	140 –170	170 –180	180 –190	190+	N/A	N/A	200
21–25	<135	135 –165	165 –175	175 –185	185+	N/A	N/A	195
26–30	<130	130 –160	160 –170	170 –180	180+	N/A	N/A	190
31–35	<125	125 –155	155 –165	165 –175	175+	N/A	N/A	185
36–40	<120	120 –150	150 –160	160 –170	170+	N/A	N/A	180
41–45	<113	115 –145	145 –155	155 –165	165+	N/A	N/A	175
46–50	<110	110 –140	140 –150	150 –160	160+	N/A	N/A	170
51–55	<105	105 –135	135 –145	145 –155	155+	N/A	N/A	165
56–60	<100	100 –130	130 –140	140 –150	150+	N/A	N/A	160
61–65	<95	95 –125	125 –135	135 –145	145+	N/A	N/A	155
66–70	<90	90 –120	120 –130	130 –140	140+	N/A	N/A	150
71–75	<85	85 –115	115 –125	125 –135	135+	N/A	N/A	145
76–80	<80	80 –110	110 –130	120 –130	130+	N/A	N/A	140
81–85	<75	75 –105	105 –115	115 –125	125+	N/A	N/A	135
86–90	<70	70 –100	100 –110	110 –120	120+	N/A	N/A	130

* Through prediction.

FEMALE

AGE	LD			SM	HI			*HR MAX
	AR (R)	LSD (AFL)	UT (HA)	AT (AT)	ES (RLZ)	IS	PWR	
15–20	<145	145 –175	175 –185	185 –195	195+	N/A	N/A	211
21–25	<140	140 –170	170 –180	180 –190	190+	N/A	N/A	206
26–30	<135	135 –165	165 –175	175 –185	185+	N/A	N/A	201
31–35	<130	130 –160	160 –170	170 –180	180+	N/A	N/A	196
36–40	<125	125 –155	155 –165	165 –175	175+	N/A	N/A	191
41–45	<120	120 –150	150 –160	160 –170	170+	N/A	N/A	186
46–50	<115	115 –145	145 –155	155 –165	165+	N/A	N/A	181
51–55	<110	110 –140	140 –150	150 –160	160+	N/A	N/A	176
56–60	<105	105 –135	135 –145	145 –155	155+	N/A	N/A	171
61–65	<100	100 –130	130 –140	140 –150	150+	N/A	N/A	166
66–70	<95	95 –125	125 –135	135 –145	145+	N/A	N/A	161
71–75	<90	90 –120	120 –130	130 –140	140+	N/A	N/A	156

76–80	<85	85–115	115–125	125–135	135+	N/A	N/A	151
81–85	<80	80–110	110–130	120–130	130+	N/A	N/A	146
86–90	<75	75–105	105–115	115–125	125+	N/A	N/A	141

* Through prediction (male is 220 − age, female is 226 − age).

NOTE: These are estimated, not individualised. They may not feel like the descriptions stated. If so, they are not correct; to reassess use method 2.

Fitness/fat loss training zones: R = recovery zone, AFL = aerobic/fat loss zone, HA = high aerobic zone, AT = anaerobic threshold zone, RLZ = red line zone.

Heart rates calculated on: HI heart rate is above AT. 85–95% of HR^{max} to get AT, UT is a 10-beat range below AT and LSD is 30 beats below.

Method 2: Assessing training intensities through calculation and testing—advanced method
(For experienced athletes)

You need to assess three areas (you can leave out the maximum heart rate test if you like). These are resting heart rate, maximum heart rate, and anaerobic threshold (Conconi test).

Assessing resting heart rate

By assessing your heart rate each morning for a week or two, you will be able to establish your average resting heart rate.

Take your heart rate in bed, lying down, upon waking. If you wake to an alarm, this can raise your heart rate slightly, so rest for two to three minutes before taking it. Make allowances if you have a busy day ahead (anxiety) or if you need to urinate, as both may elevate heart rate slightly. This is particularly important during a 'test' week.

Note your resting heart rate:

NOTE: if you are keen to get going, take a 'one off' resting heart rate now to get started and go back to do the tests properly later.

Calculating or testing for maximum heart rate

Maximum heart rate (HR^{max}) is the highest heart rate that you can achieve. This obviously occurs at maximum intensity or effort. Maximum heart rates can vary from 130–220 beats per minute, depending on the athlete.

CALCULATING MAXIMUM HEART RATE (THE EASY WAY)

Do the following calculation:

Male: 220 - age

Female: 226 - age

Maximum Heart Rate:

This method is easy to use but not as accurate as testing.

TESTING FOR MAXIMUM HEART RATE (THE HARD BUT ACCURATE WAY)

Taking your heart rate to maximum is completely safe unless you have a heart abnormality. If you do have a heart abnormality, be warned: a maximum heart rate test can result in death! If you are simply unfit, a maximum heart rate test can still make you feel very unwell (dizzy or nauseous).

If possible, then, acquire some cardiovascular fitness before under-

Resting heart rate should be taken in bed.

going this test. If you do this, you will find that a maximum heart rate test is not anywhere near as bad as it sounds. A fit athlete can 'hit' maximum heart rate without any damaging effects — it just doesn't feel very comfortable. The American College of Sports Medicine has this to say about maximum heart rate tests:

> *At or above 35 years of age, it is necessary for individuals to have a medical examination and a maximal exercise test before beginning a vigorous exercise programme. At any age, the information gathered from an exercise test may be useful to establish an effective and safe exercise prescription. Maximal testing done for men at age 40 or above, and women at age 50 or above, even when no symptoms or risk factors are present, should be performed with physician supervision.*

The safest way to assess maximum heart rate is to get a doctor or sports physiologist to do a stress test and conduct a health appraisal. The test can be conducted safely and precisely to indicate maximum heart rate.

The test will also provide other interesting information:

- Resting heart function (ECG).
- Exercise and maximum heart function (ECG).
- Rest/exercise blood pressures.
- Anaerobic threshold (LT or VE).
- Aerobic threshold.
- Projected approximate training and racing speeds.

These tests cost between $50 and $200 and are available through most exercise testing labs.

The other way to go is to do a self-administered maximum heart rate test. But consider getting a testing lab to determine your maximum heart rate if:

- You are over 35 years of age.
- You have been sedentary (inactive) for over 12 months.
- You have never had a maximum heart rate test before, or have not exercised close to maximal exertion in the last 12 months.
- You are in poor physical condition.

If you are in poor physical condition, have a complete physical check-up by a doctor and don't exercise until your doctor has cleared you to do so.

If none of the above apply, you are almost ready to do a self-administered maximum heart rate test.

Preparation for HR^{max} tests

Do not eat for 2–3 hours before a HR^{max} test. If you do, you may feel nauseous or have stomach cramps during or after the test. Always warm up and warm down for your tests.

Safety

If, during the test, you feel either dizzy or nauseous, want to stop, have chest pain or numbness down your left arm, have difficulty breathing, or your heart rate monitor gives unusually high or fluctuating readings, reduce intensity immediately (below 100 beats per minute) and stop the test.

Keep pedalling (or jogging) lightly, however, so you don't get dizzy and pass out. Consult a doctor as soon as possible. If during the test your heart rate goes above the age-adjusted formula (220 minus your age for men; 226 minus your age for women) be a little cautious. Do not do the test if you have a cold or other illness.

Self-administered maximum heart rate tests

To find your maximum heart rate, warm up for 10–15 minutes. Once warmed up, exercise as hard you can for 4–8 minutes, with the last 1–2 minutes at maximum effort, until you 'blow'!

Your maximum heart rate is the highest reliable heart rate reached during testing on the road or a stationary trainer— your 'high score'. This is best worked out using a heart rate monitor, but you can work it out manually as long as you manage to take your heart rate immediately after the test.

Maximum heart rate: ☐

TROUBLE-SHOOTING MAXIMUM HEART RATE TESTS

For specific information on trouble-shooting, see *Precision Training*.

As a simple check, calculate maximum theoretical heart rate by using the formula 220 minus age for men or 226 minus age for women.

Assessing anaerobic threshold — Conconi test

This test is very strenuous! Get medical clearance if you are unsure about your ability to cope with it, particularly if you are over the age of 35.

The advantage of the Conconi test is that it is very simple, does not require a lot of expensive testing equipment and, with the help of a couple of assistants, you can conduct it yourself. You will need:

- an accurate heart rate monitor.

- an assistant to record heart rates/lap splits.

- a bike equipped with a computer to measure speed and cadence.

- a velodrome (choose a windless day) or a stationary cycle trainer.

For testing other sports, see *The Power to Perform* or *Precision Training*.

THE TEST

Warm up for 10–20 minutes. Each lap should be between 300 and 450 m for a velodrome test. If you use your wind-trainer, use an appropriate time interval (30 seconds between speed increases).

In the velodrome test, ride and maintain constant pace and cadence during each lap. Increase your speed by 1 or 2 kph each lap (use the same increase each lap) until your legs are too tired to continue. At the end of each lap call out your heart rate and speed so that it can be recorded by your assistant (using the sheet on page 39). For the stationary trainer test, start at around 100 watts for an experienced athlete and increase the load by 10/20 watts every 30 seconds (10 watts for beginners, 20 watts if experienced). Record wattage and heart rate for each load.

See appendix 3 for other aspects you can combine in this test.

HOW TO CALCULATE ANAEROBIC THRESHOLD

Calculate your speed (cycling) per section of lap for velodrome tests — stationary trainer tests don't require this (see page 39). Plot your results on the graph on page 40, charting your recorded heart rates on the vertical axis and your speed/watts on the horizontal axis. If your test has gone as planned, your graph should show an evenly sloping upward line until the point where your heart rate was unable to increase at the same rate as speed (heart rate plateau). The heart rate at this heart rate plateau 'deflection point' is your anaerobic threshold heart rate (see fig 4.1).

HOW OFTEN DO YOU NEED TO TEST?

Anaerobic threshold can move, so you need to test it regularly. AT should improve (get higher) during speedwork (see fig 4.2).

Test every 2–8 weeks, towards the end of an easy week in your programme. Rest for 18–24 hours before the test to freshen up. Test every two weeks in the Speed phase and every eight weeks in the Base phase. Try to keep test conditions identical so that you get accurate results.

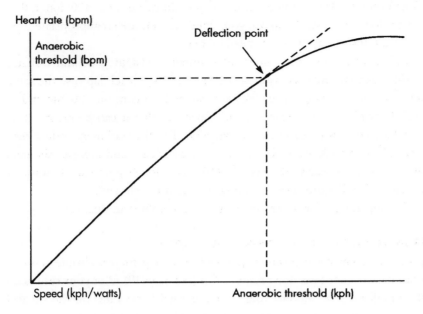

Fig 4.1: Anaerobic threshold test (Conconi), showing heart rate vs speed

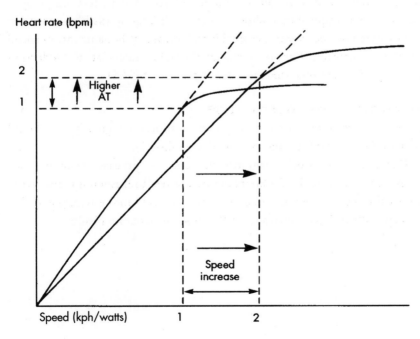

Fig 4.2: Change in anaerobic threshold (heart rate and speed) at the start of speedwork (1) and after peak (2)

Conconi test record sheet

Name: Date:

LAP	HEART RATE	TIME (SECS/LAP)	SPEED/WATTAGE

Speed calculations in kph:

As above for lap time and ap distance

Lap distance (km) ÷ lap time (mins) x 60 = speed (kph)

LAP	HEART RATE	TIME (SECS/LAP)	SPEED/WATTAGE
1.	....	....	....
2.	....	....	....
3.	....	....	....
4.	....	....	....
5.	....	....	....
6.	....	....	....
7.	....	....	....
8.	....	....	....
9.	....	....	....
10.	....	....	....
11.	....	....	....
12.	....	....	....
13.	....	....	....
14.	....	....	....
15.	....	....	....
16.	....	....	....
17.	....	....	....
18.	....	....	....
19.	....	....	....
20.	....	....	....

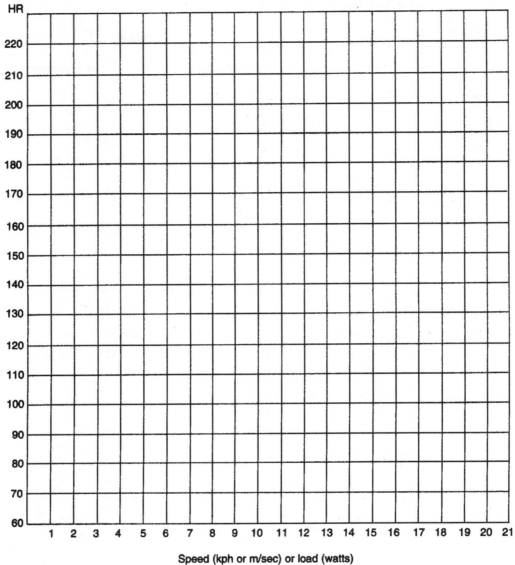

Speed (kph or m/sec) or load (watts)

Test duration: ....

Fig 4.3: Anaerobic/aerobic threshold assessment sheet

Anaerobic threshold heart rate: ☐

To calculate training heart rates:

1. Take your AT heart rate and round it to the nearest 5 beats:
   e.g. 183 = 185.

2. Subtract and add 5 beats to give a range:
   e.g. 180–190.

3. Subtract 10 beats from the bottom of your SM range to give the bottom of your UT range:
   e.g. 180 - 10 = 170; UT = 170–180

4. Use the Karvonen formula at 60% to get the bottom of your LSD range:
   e.g. (204 - 45) x 60% + 45 = 140

5. The top of your AT heart rate to maximum heart rate is HI:
   e.g. 190–204

6. AR is the bottom of the LSD range or less (e.g. <140).

Put rates in the tables provided in the 'Putting it all together' section below.

Putting it all together

○ Put all your heart rates in.

Karvonen formula

$(HR^{max} – HR^{rest})$ x (% exercise intensity) + HR^{rest}

HR^{max} = maximum heart rate; HR^{rest} = resting heart rate.

Maximum heart rate: ☐

(assessed either by physical test or 220 – age [males]; 226 – age [females]).

Threshold heart rate: ☐

(by test or ignore)

Resting heart rate: ☐

(taken lying down in bed on waking)

HIGH INTENSITY (ANAEROBIC)/RED LINE ZONE

INTENSITY	DURATION	%HR^{MAX}
Power	Less than 10 sec	N/A
Intensive sprints	10 sec–1 min	N/A
Extensive sprints	1–4 min	95–100%

(HI)/(RLZ)

SUBMAXIMAL INTENSITY (THRESHOLD)/ANAEROBIC THRESHOLD

INTENSITY	DURATION	%HR^{MAX}
Maximum steady-state pace	4 min–1 hr	N/A
Anaerobic threshold	1 hr	85–95%

(AT)/(AT)

LOW INTENSITY (AEROBIC/HIGH AEROBIC/FAT LOSS & RECOVERY) ZONE

INTENSITY	DURATION	%HR^{MAX}
Up-tempo	4 min+	75–85%

(UT)/(HA)

INTENSITY	DURATION	%HR^{MAX}
Long Slow distance	4 min+	60–75%

(LSD)/(AFL)

Active recovery	4 min+	<60%

(AR)/(R)

NOTE: For calculated heart rates rather than assessed, it is impossible to obtain absolutely accurate training heart rate ranges. These percentages are designed to give you an approximate level to train in, and using the training intensity descriptions you should be able to establish your training levels accurately by heart rate and by feel.

In short intervals it is difficult to use heart rates as they may not react fast enough. For sprints it is recommended that you use the specified durations. For tempo and anaerobic threshold intervals, it will take 1–3 mins for your heart rate to 'react' to changes in intensity. Do the interval at the pace you feel is correct and let the heart rate slowly come up to confirm it.

Bike and stationary trainer specifics

The stationary trainer

Road vs trainer workouts

Generally, training on the road is better than training using a stationary trainer because training involves showing your body what happens on race day — in other words, simulating race conditions and intensities. Riding on the road teaches balance, gear changing to suit the terrain, and many other skills that cannot be learnt on a stationary trainer. On the other hand, if you go out each night in the cold, the rain and the dark you will probably lose your enthusiasm (obviously winter is the big test), and you may be playing 'bicycle roulette' with your health. A balance is therefore necessary.

Often athletes will do one or two (sometimes all) of their work-day sessions on their stationary trainer. These tend to be shorter sessions, and often speed sessions, as these can be very effective on a trainer. Road rides are completed on the weekend, and these are generally longer sessions. Avoid doing long sessions on your trainer; mentally it's very tough. They drive me nuts! My limit is 2 hours, although I have heard of athletes who do 6-hour rides on their trainer. Ugh!!

So what do you do if you substitute a trainer workout for a road ride because there is a force-10 hurricane blowing outside?

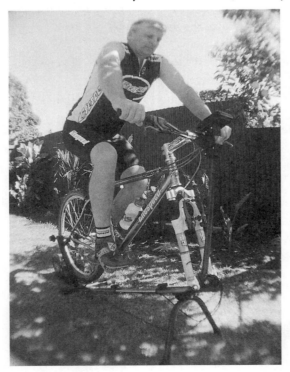

Spinning outside can be a happy compromise between indoor training and road rides.

Stationary trainer myths and mistakes

- The general reaction seems to be to abandon the scheduled workout, jump on the trainer and do a short session full of intervals. What effect does that have on your training? You plan your training and your workout carefully, and then you change it because you are on a stationary trainer. A stationary trainer or cyclosimulator is just that — it simulates training that you would do on the road. So whatever you were supposed to do on the road you should do on the trainer.

- How to overtrain on a stationary trainer! As we have discussed, the tendency on trainers is to do short workouts with lots of intervals. If you do this on the road more than 2 or 3 times a week you'll burn out within 3–5 weeks. Surprisingly enough, the same thing happens on your stationary trainer. There are more methods of training than just doing intervals on your trainer.

- Now here's a myth. A stationary trainer workout is twice as hard as a road workout so you only have to do half as much! Stationary trainers are hard for several reasons — we'll mention them in a second. To convert your road training to your stationary trainer, reduce the duration by about 10 percent to allow for freewheeling (a 120-minute ride on the road equals a 108-minute ride on your trainer) and alternate some standing with sitting to give the muscles a bit of a rest.

How to make life easier on a stationary trainer (becoming a stationary trainer 'leisure master')

Let's face it, stationary trainers aren't the most comfortable things around.

- They're boring.

- You can't freewheel down the hills.

- You are seated the whole time.

- Your legs get tired because you move around less on a trainer, 'burning out' the areas of the muscle you are working in the riding position.

- There is no wind to cool you off. On the road the wind passing over your body causes sweat to evaporate and this cools you down. On a stationary trainer there is no wind blowing over you, so the sweat doesn't evaporate and your body begins to heat up. When your body core temperature heats up even slightly, this impairs performance. But you don't necessarily feel hot, you feel grotty.

So let's make things as comfortable as possible. Let's get the 'leisure' bit right. If you can master at least three remotes to control major household appliances (preferably TV/Sky decoder, video and CD player) you are a 'leisure master'. This means that you know how to relax using the full range of 1990s technology.

To become a 'leisure master':

- Get a really big fan to keep you cool.
- Get a really big TV (26-inch plus) with Sky decoder and remote (within arm's reach of course).
- Get a really big multiple CD player with remote (again, within arm's reach of course).
- Have a really good emergency back-up walkman with tapes and spare batteries at arm's reach.
- Get a really big video player with remote (within arm's reach of course) — suggested videos are the Tour de France, Hawaii Ironman and Mammoth Mountain Downhill (long versions).
- Get a really big fluffy towel to dry the sweat and a mat on the floor to catch the drips.
- Here's the biggie — convince your partner, wife, live-in lover or flat-mates that it is not only okay but highly necessary that you train in front of the aforementioned appliances.

    (Also mention that the volumes on the various appliances need to be very high so that you can hear over the noise of the stationary trainer and can experience the full atmosphere of 'being there'.)
- Bonus points can be achieved by training in the living room (to go to the garage to train is to suffer terribly) and by keeping your bike stored inside the house.

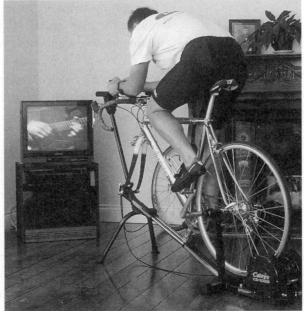

A good TV or sound system are the main tools for becoming a leisure master.

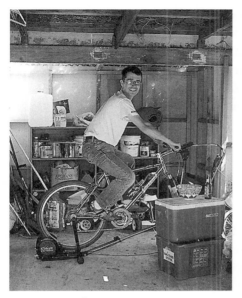

How not to do it

Once you have reached these lofty heights you can officially call yourself a 'leisure master' and say that you have a 'Masters in Leisure'. Your stationary training will be pleasure itself and the results in terms of performance will be excellent.

Seriously, some of the aforementioned hints are worth noting as they will make indoor training more bearable.

Important points for stationary trainers

• Drape towels over your trainer where the sweat falls. This prevents rusting and stops sweat getting all over the floor/carpet.

• Buy a plastic mat to put under the trainer so that bicycle grease and rubber off the tyres don't get on the floor or stain the carpet.

• Watch for frame flex, which can weaken or bend your beautiful racing frame. In most cases this is not a problem, but it is a risk for cyclists using a very light racing frame who are muscularly very strong. If you are worried ask a coach, your local cycle shop or an experienced cyclist about it.

• Keep your trainer calibrated so you can see improvements in testing and in training.

The bike

Gears and how they work

There are two major geared areas on a bike. The first is the chainrings or chainwheels, which are at the front of the bike. The second area is the rear sprockets or cluster. Both areas contain different sized sprockets with teeth on them.

CHAINRINGS

Chainrings are the large cogs on the front of the bike near the pedals. They control the gross changes in resistance in the gears. There are two chainrings on a racing cycle, while mountain bikes have three. Chainrings are defined by the number of teeth they have; for example, if a chainring has 42 teeth, it is usually called a '42'. Common chainrings on racing bikes are 52/39, 52/42 and 53/42. This is the number of teeth on each chainring. So 52/42 means 52 teeth on the big chainring and 42 teeth on the smaller chainring. Mountain bikes usually have 22/32/42 to 22/34/36 chainring combinations. The larger the chainring the higher the resistance as this means it takes more distance to 'roll out' one pedal revolution. The chainring is selected by adjusting the gear levers that cause the front derailleur to move the chain.

REAR SPROCKETS

Rear sprockets control the finer, more subtle changes to gearing on the bike. They are also defined by the number of teeth. Common cluster ranges are from 12–21. This means the bike has 12-, 13-, 14-, 15-, 16-, 17-, 18-, and 21-tooth sprockets or a similar progression. Unlike chainrings, where the more teeth the chainring has the higher the resistance, the more teeth a rear sprocket has the lower the resistance. This is because the bigger the chainring at the front and the smaller the chainring at the back the more 'roll out' you have to turn over one pedal revolution. The bigger the cog at the back the easier the gear will be, and you will have less 'rollout' (distance to cover in the course of one complete pedal revolution). The rear sprockets are selected by adjusting the gear levers that cause the rear derailleur to move the chain.

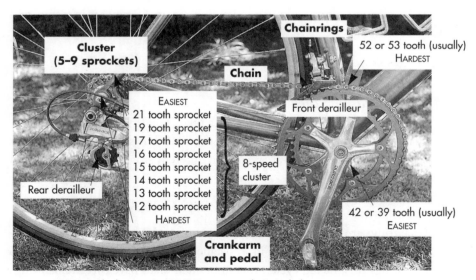

52 (52-tooth chainring) x 17 (17-gear sprocket) *might be your racing gear*

Fig. 5.1: The drive chain — cycle gearing system

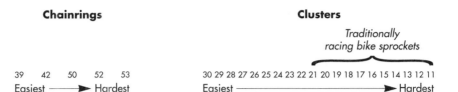

Chainrings

39 42 50 52 53

Easiest ⟶ Hardest

Clusters

Traditionally racing bike sprockets

30 29 28 27 26 25 24 23 22 21 20 19 18 17 16 15 14 13 12 11

Easiest ⟶ Hardest

Fig. 5.2: The ratio between the front chain ring and the rear sprockets provide a gear number (road cycle example)

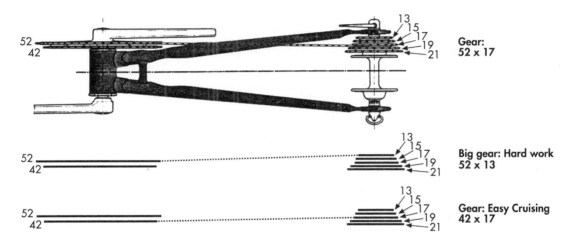

Fig. 5.3: The easy and hard of gears

Chainring x rear sprocket — putting them together

Cycling terminology describes the resistance used or required on the bike in terms of gears — chainring x rear sprocket (for example, 42 x 18). A 53 x 12 is a very big gear (big cog at the front and little cog at the back — big x little); a 52 x 21 or 42 x 12 are medium gears (big x big; little x little), while a very small gear might be a 42 x 21 (little x big).

If this all seems confusing don't worry; as you use your bike more and more you will soon get used to the terminology (see fig 5.3).

Knowing your gears

Count the number of teeth on each chainring and sprocket on your rear cluster so that you know what all your gears are:

CHAINRING	CLUSTER (SPROCKETS)
1. ———————	1. ———————
2. ———————	2. ———————
3. ——————— (for MTB)	3. ———————
	4. ———————
	5. ———————
	6. ———————
	7. ———————
	8. ———————
	9. ———————

Cadence

Cadence is the number of revolutions a pedal will complete in one minute. Common cadences are around 85–95 rpm for time trials, mountain biking, triathlons, duathlons and time-trial-type multisport events, and 95–105 rpm for cycle racing and triathlons and multisport events that require drafting (slip-streaming off other cyclists to reduce air resistance and save energy). The reason cadence is higher for cycle racing is that if someone sprints off up the road you need to be able to speed up quickly to catch them, which a high cadence allows you to do. If you have a low cadence you have to wind the gear up, which takes too much time and effort. In time-trialling you hold a constant pace and there aren't sudden accelerations, so it is more efficient physiologically and biomechanically to use a lower cadence and push a bigger gear. Cadences don't have to be that high on the hills; they generally drop down to 40–60 rpm.

OPTIMAL PEDAL CADENCES

For triathlon, duathlon, mountain biking and time trials: 85–95 rpm.
For cycle racing and multisport races in bunches: 90–105 rpm.

Variations:

- Older (vet and masters) athletes are usually more comfortable at the lower ends of the ranges.
- Stronger athletes tend to be at the lower ends of the ranges, with weaker cyclists at the upper end.
- Fitter athletes tend to be at the higher ends of the ranges, while less fit athletes tend to be at the lower end.

Training on the bike and stationary trainer

Correcting strength/strength endurance imbalances

The difference between strength and strength endurance is that strength is the ability to move a resistance (e.g. pedal revolutions) up to, say, 20 times, while strength endurance is the ability to move a resistance up to 500 or so times.

Strength and strength endurance imbalances between legs can cause injuries, as well as affect technique and performance. They often occur as a result of past injuries which lead to a favouring of one leg, and sometimes as a consequence of back trouble. Strength/strength endurance imbalances often lead to overuse injuries as the weaker leg becomes overtrained in comparison with the stronger leg, and back problems can also arise due to the unequal power being generated by the legs.

Technique can become affected as it is adjusted to compensate for the injury, and performance also suffers as the weaker leg is delivering less power and is not maintaining the momentum of the power generated by the stronger leg.

How to test for strength/strength endurance imbalances

- Warm up for 10–20 minutes on the stationary trainer (with several efforts at high resistance).
- Put the bike in a large gear (52 x 12–15) or put a high gradient (7–10 percent) on the stationary trainer.
- Remove one leg from the pedal binding and place it in the bottom bracket 'v' created by the down tube and the seat tube.
- Pedal with one leg for a 10- to 15-second sprint then subjectively assess

your level of muscular fatigue, or pedal at 50–60 rpm until you cannot complete another pedal revolution and count how many full revolutions you completed on that leg (you must use the same method if you repeat the test at a later date).

- Rest to recovery by spinning in a small gear with both legs for a few minutes.
- Repeat the procedure using the other leg.
- Test 2–3 times, alternating the legs.
- Warm down for 5–10 minutes.

A definite subjective indication that there is a strength difference between legs, or a noticeable difference between the numbers of repetitions completed on each leg, indicates a strength imbalance. Another indicator is an increased amount of wear on your seat on the side of the weaker leg.

You can test for general strength imbalances on weight training equipment but testing yourself on your bike, while it may not seem as accurate, is specific to your cycling strength. You may have balanced general strength, but not cycling strength.

Correcting strength imbalances using your stationary trainer

- Warm up for 10 minutes on the stationary trainer (with several efforts at high resistance).
- Put the bike in a large gear (52 x 12–15) or put a high gradient (7–10 percent) on the stationary trainer.
- Remove the stronger leg from the pedal binding and place it in the bottom bracket 'v' created by the seat tube and the down tube.
- Cycle on the weaker leg for periods of 20 seconds to 5 minutes (20 seconds to 1 minute for strength; 1 to 5 minutes for strength endurance).
- Rest for 3–4 times the work period for strength training, and for twice the work period for strength endurance training. Spin in an easy gear with both legs during your rest period.
- Do this anywhere between 3 and 10 times.
- Warm down for 10–15 minutes, concentrating on technique.
- If you do this as part of another workout, do it at the end of the workout. Do this 2–4 times per week on a day-on, day-off basis for a period of 6–8 weeks, then retest. If you are having trouble getting results, see a reputable

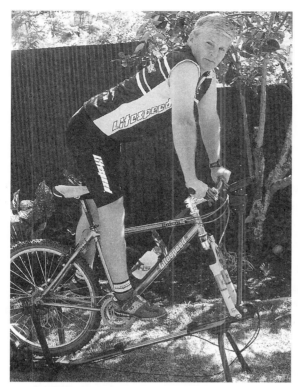

A mountain bike or racing bike is equally good for spinning, but in both cases varying leg position helps to achieve a full workout.

coach or a strength training expert and add strength training using weight training equipment. You should usually correct strength imbalances in the off-season as it can be harmful to your training performance and make you susceptible to injury in your training and competition periods. This is because a weak leg is generally more fatigued by training; to fatigue it further by doing strength imbalance correction exercises can lead to overuse injuries. Correct strength imbalances when the training volumes are low and the intensity is not high (see page 167).

Technique training

Why do technique?

Most cyclists do not use their leg muscles to the full extent in terms of delivering power to the pedals. The more effective the leg muscles are and the more they are used, the more power you can generate and the faster you can go.

A lot of cyclists only push down on the pedals, while others only push down and pull up. The key is to generate power throughout the whole pedal stroke, thus retaining through the whole stroke the momentum that is produced by the powerful down-stroke.

Additional equipment

You need a mirror to see your cycling technique (front and side if possible), and a music stand to hold this book, a magazine or a novel.

The cycling action

The cycling action can be broken down into four major parts:

- The down-stroke — the quadriceps (front of the thigh) are the main muscles used in the down-stroke, followed by the gluteal muscles (buttocks) near the bottom of the stroke.

- Bottom of the stroke — the gluteals are still used at the start of the back-stroke, followed by the calves which give a 'pushing down' to toe-pointing action in the middle of the bottom of the back-stroke, and towards the end of the back-stroke the hamstrings (backs of the thighs) begin to pull back and the muscles at the front of the shin begin to pull up so that the toe points up again.

- The up-stroke — the hamstrings continue to pull up but the shin muscles stop as the toe is now pointed up. Close to the top of the up-stroke the powerful hip muscles (the hip flexors) begin to contribute to pulling up.

- Top of the stroke — the hamstrings phase out and the hip flexors drive the pedal to the top of the stroke causing the knees to come up, and finally, just after the top of the stroke, the big quadriceps muscles phase in to begin the down-stroke.

So there it is — not quite as simple as putting one foot in front of the other.

Now how do you go about developing your technique? The following exercises will help. Start with the first ones, then move on to the more advanced exercises as you improve.

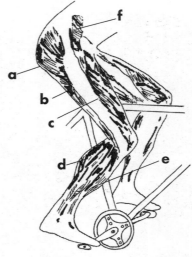

Fig. 6.1: Some of the major leg muscles used in cycling: the gluteal (buttock) muscles (a), hamstrings (b), quadriceps (c), calf muscle (d), tibialis anterior (shin) (e), and hip flexor (f).

1. Spinning — riding at the correct cadence

Triathlon, duathlon, mountain biking and time trialling require pedal cadences of 85–95 rpm. Cycle racing and triathlon with legal drafting require cadences of around 95–105 rpm.

Most beginners tend to ride at too low a cadence, while older cyclists particularly tend to find it difficult to 'spin'. To rectify this, spin training can be used. This involves pedalling in a very easy gear (39 or 42 x 17–21) at the required cadence. You can either use a cycle computer which has cadence as a monitoring function or count the number of pedal revolutions one leg does in 30 seconds and double this figure. For example, 45 pedal revolutions in 30 seconds = 45 x 2 = 90 rpm.

The key factors are to stay in a small to very small gear so you are not hammering, and to try to relax as you spin.

2. Fluidity of pedalling

Downhill spinning sprints can be used to enhance your fluidity of pedalling. This teaches you to ride in circles not squares. Cycling in squares means either only pushing down on the pedals or only pushing down and pulling up. Cycling in circles means pushing down, pulling back, pulling up and pulling over on the pedals. By cycling in circles you apply force through the full circle of a pedal revolution. The advantages are that you are more relaxed, conserve energy as you spread the load around more muscles, and are faster because you use more muscles and maintain momentum through each pedal revolution. The bottom line is you go faster for longer for less effort.

Spinning is everything when it comes to cycling. Spinning is your ability to pedal through a full range of pedal motions with optimum speed and fluidity. One way to check whether you are achieving this is to listen to your stationary trainer. If the sound rises and falls with each pedal revolution you know that you are not spinning. The sound changes because the flywheel or roller increases in speed as you push harder, increasing the sound, and the sound decreases as the force you apply drops. Often the sound is loudest when you push down. If you are spinning the sound should remain constant. The change can be heard best at lower pedal cadences.

Make sure you check not only your seated spinning but your standing spinning. A lot of people spin well seated but spin badly when they stand up.

To conduct downhill or flat spinning sprints put your bike in a little gear (39 or 42 x 18–21) and aim to achieve around 120–150 pedal revolutions for around 30 seconds to 1 minute. Do 1–6 intervals of this.

You will find that as you increase the cadence to higher revolutions you will start to bounce around on your seat. This is because you are not relaxing your muscles fast enough. In other words, some muscles are contracting to apply force on the pedals before other muscles have relaxed fully. This causes a jerky pedalling action which makes you bounce around. What you do is increase pedal cadence until this occurs then try to relax your legs to stop the bouncing.

As you practise this you will find that your muscles will learn the 'firing pattern' of the cycling movement and your pedalling will become more fluid and relaxed.

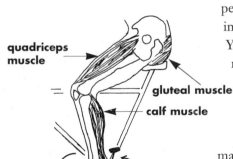

quadriceps
muscle

gluteal muscle

calf muscle

Fig. 6.2: The muscles used in the bottom of the pedal stroke

3. 'Scraping mud off your shoe' — bottom of the pedal stroke

This is to improve your ability to work through the bottom of the pedal stroke. The action is very similar to scraping mud off your shoe, in that it is a pushing down, pulling back action. The idea is to work on this action through the bottom of the pedal stroke.

4. Pulling up — the up-stroke

This action is relatively straightforward. The pulling up is simply pulling the pedal back and up to maintain the momentum and power of the strong down-stroke. Try to feel the hamstrings at the back of the thigh contracting to pull the pedal back to the top of the stroke.

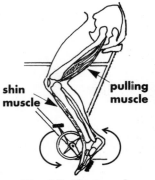

Fig. 6.3: The muscles used in the up-stroke

5. 'Up and kick the door' — top of the pedal stroke

The aim of this exercise is to simulate lifting your knee up then to 'kick the door'. The action therefore comes from the hip first, then from the quadriceps for the 'kicking' action. This means that as your leg reaches a position 20–30 degrees before the top of the pedal stroke you use your hips (hip flexors) to pull the pedal to the top of the stroke. As the pedal reaches the top of the stroke the quadriceps (front of the thighs) initiate the beginnings of the push down for the start of the down-stroke.

Be careful and start gradually, as overemphasising this training too suddenly can cause knee problems. This is generally the worst trained area of the pedal stroke in most cyclists so it's an area that merits some effort.

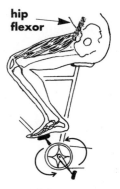

Fig. 6.4: The muscles used in the top of the pedal stroke

6. Pushing down — the down-stroke

This area doesn't rate any real technique training as new cyclists tend to focus on it naturally, and it's an area of strength for most cyclists (see fig 6.5).

7. Combinations — up and down, over and back

Now that you have mastered each isolated action or technique, you want to combine them. Here are two useful exercises.

a. To combine the up-stroke and the down-stroke, focus on the down-stroke of one leg while working on the up-stroke on the other leg. Both legs are therefore producing the power through different actions at the same time. Concentrate on the right down/left up combination for 10–30 pedal strokes, then on the left down/right up combination. You'll generally find that one leg will require more work than the other.

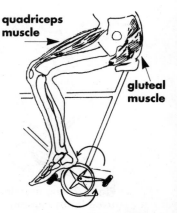

Fig. 6.5: The muscles used in the down-stroke

b. The other combination is to work over the top of the pedal stroke and the bottom of the pedal stroke in left leg over/right leg back and right leg over/left leg back combinations in a similar fashion to above.

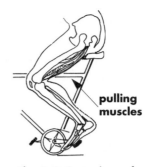

pulling muscles

Fig. 6.6: Experienced cyclists use more muscles for spinning.

8. Working through the whole pedal stroke —Big gear/little gear

A lot of cyclists do not apply force through the whole pedal stroke. There are inherent problems with this as biomechanically it is difficult to do through the bottom and top of a pedal revolution. Obviously this is a weak area.

To improve this a high-resistance exercise can be used, but you need to be careful and condition yourself by doing several weeks of spinning sprints before doing this, as you can injure your knees. Athletes under 16 years of age or those with past knee problems should not do this exercise.

The exercise is performed for no more than 1 minute for each interval and the resistance is high enough that you can barely turn the gears over. The effect is that because the resistance is so high you learn to apply force throughout the entire pedal revolution just to keep pedalling — if force is not applied throughout the full pedal stroke you will be unable to keep pedalling. You can do some 'transfer' training by alternating the big gear efforts with little gear spinning sprints.

9. Knees in and correcting the wobble

KNEES IN

Athletes who have tight iliotibial bands (the tendon on the outside of the thighs) and sometimes tight gluteal muscles (buttocks) and lower back often pedal with their knees pointed out. This is a weak position in terms of delivering power to the pedals.

If you see this sort of pedalling action in your mirror when doing technique (particularly when you get tired) get a doctor, physio or massage therapist to check whether you are tight in that area. Also get an experienced cycle coach or cyclist to check your pedal alignment specific to you.

If you are tight then get massage or do stretches, and if necessary get your pedal alignment set up properly, then start working on bringing your knees in. Don't fight it though, as you may cause injury.

If you are not tight it may be that you are biomechanically and naturally supposed to be this way. In this case consult a sports podiatrist regarding what you should do. If possible, though, the most powerful position is to have your knees over the pedals.

CORRECTING THE WOBBLE

Some cyclists' knees only point out at the top of the pedal stroke but realign correctly on the down-stroke and up-stroke. This creates a wobble through the pedalling stroke and can predispose the athlete to knee injuries. This is far more likely to be the result of a tight iliotibial band, gluteal muscles or tight lower back. Follow the same recommendations as for 'knees in'.

Artificial heat acclimatisation using a stationary trainer

Using your stationary trainer in the right conditions can be a good way of acclimatising your body when you are planning to compete in the heat. Any athlete competing in an environment that is not conducive to heat loss is at risk of heat injury and a drop in performance.

When travelling to any country where ambient temperature is above 25.6°C, acclimatisation is necessary. It takes between 7 and 10 days to acclimatise to hot, humid climates. Even if the temperature is below 25.6°C, but hotter than where you normally train, some form of acclimatisation is advisable.

To heat acclimatise you can either train in a hot environment or you can artificially heat acclimatise on your stationary trainer.

The key to acclimatisation is to get used to exercising in the heat. It is not good enough to simply live in the hot environment — you must train in the heat (same environmental conditions, same training intensity and a similar training duration). If you race in the middle of the day and it is very hot, you need to be conditioned to racing in that kind of environment. The exercise intensity should be at least 70–75 percent of VO_{2max} to evoke adaptation (heart rate at 155–160 bpm for a 25-year-old).

Temperature and humidity

It is important to understand the relationship between temperature and humidity. Temperatures up to 25°C are safe even in high humidity. However, when the temperature climbs to 27°C an increase in humidity can be very dangerous.

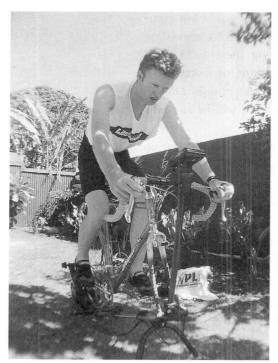

Train in the heat to get used to a hot environment.

High humidity (water vapour in the air) will not allow adequate evaporation of sweat from the body. Sweating is the body's way of reducing its core temperature. If the core temperature gets too high, you begin to experience the first symptoms of heat stress. If it continues to climb, you may suffer from potentially fatal heat injury.

To get used to a hot environment, you need to train in the heat. To get used to a hot, humid environment you need to train in the heat and the humidity. Many athletes have made the mistake of adapting to the heat but not the humidity. This can be dangerous.

Other factors

Temperature and humidity are not the only contributing factors to heat stress. Others include lack of sleep, infection and glycogen depletion.

It is a good idea in hot climates to weigh yourself before and after workouts to keep a check on fluid loss. Any weight loss is fluid loss! Drink one litre of fluid for every kilogram of bodyweight lost during exercise.

A 2 percent loss in bodyweight after a workout or race (1.4 kg loss for a 70-kg athlete) represents a fluid loss due to thermal or exercise-induced dehydration. This decreases muscular strength and endurance considerably. Dehydration can affect training for 24 to 36 hours as it takes time to rehydrate completely. Urine colour should be clear if you are well hydrated (unless you are taking vitamin pills). Try alternating water and sport drinks to avoid losing salt and potassium.

Artificial heat acclimatisation

Artificial heat acclimatisation may be necessary if you cannot get to the competition venue early enough. This form of heat training has been carried out in heat chambers, greenhouses and heated training rooms. For many athletes, however, these may not be available.

Another technique for inducing hot conditions artificially involves wearing excessive layers of clothing while exercising, especially layers on the head. Acclimatising to hot conditions in these ways is quite often necessary for athletes living in one hemisphere and racing in another.

Alternating techniques for different workouts is acceptable but combining two techniques can overwhelm the body's temperature regulating mechanism and lead to problems. If you are using these techniques, gradually increase the heat stress (add layers of clothing or increase the room temperature) over the 7 to 10 days prior to competition. Do not overdo it! Training in the same temperature as the race will be run in is sufficient. Hotter is not better!

Finally, if you are training in a heated room, use a fan to aid evaporation of sweat from the body.

ARTIFICIAL HEAT ACCLIMATISATION

- Put a heater or two in a closed room.
- Let the room heat up for 20–40 minutes (you can use a thermometer to check the temperature).
- Do the workout on your stationary trainer in the room.

ARTIFICIAL HEAT AND HUMIDITY ACCLIMATISATION

- Follow the same directions as above.
- Drape several wet towels over a water heater in the room (as the heater dries the towels the water turns into vapour and creates humidity).

WARNING: This is not all that good for the house!

Training programmes

This chapter enables you to select your 16-week, sport-specific programme (pages 65–81). Further, you should be able to select the appropriate spinning workouts (stationary or road) for each training session or week (pages 82–146). In the training programmes that follow, more than one programme is given for each sport, taking into account the type and duration or distance of each event (check the title of each programme under 'race' in the top left corner).

Go through the sports below and find a programme that suits you. The training programmes set out in this book give you a choice of over 56 workouts across 17 programmes for 5 different sports.

Choosing your sport and programme

Sport	Pages	No. of programmes
Triathlon	65–69	5
Duathlon	70–71	2
Multisport	72–73	2
Road cycling	74–79	6
Mountain biking	80–81	2

Select the programme that suits the type of race you are aiming for (for example, within the sport of cycling you can select programmes for 40-km, 80-km, 100-km, 160-km and tour racing).

Running your programme
How far do I go?

USING THE PROGRAMME ON THE ROAD
You will see on the programmes that you have a training duration/distance for each day in minutes or kilometres. This is the length of time or distance you will

work out for if you are training on the road. (For example, in the cycling programme on page 77, for week 9, Saturday, it tells you to ride 49 km.) For multiple-sport events like triathlon it gives you the workouts for the other sports. (For example, in the triathlon programme on page 65, for week 9, Thursday, it tells you to *run* 7.2 km.)

USING THE PROGRAMME ON YOUR STATIONARY TRAINER

If you are using a stationary trainer, ignore the volumes on the programme and use the durations that are scheduled in the pre-written spinning workouts in (see chapter 8, 'Spinning workouts', pages 82–146). The following workouts will further clarify this.

What do I do?

Next to the duration/distance is a subtext number (1,2,3, etc.) which indicates the type of training (subphase) you should do. So, on page 77, for week 9 on Saturday the numbers are 49_5. You can look up this number in chapter 8, 'Spinning workouts' (pages 82–146). The subtext number (e.g. $_5$ in 49_5) that matches the number in chapter 8 gives you information on how to do the training in that workout. (For example, using the same cycling workout on page 77, the subtext number for the Saturday 49-km cycle is '5'. If you look up what to do in chapter 8, page 110, you will see this equates to up-tempo training, and there is a description of how to do that type of training. Six different specific spinning workouts are given on the pages immediately after the description.)

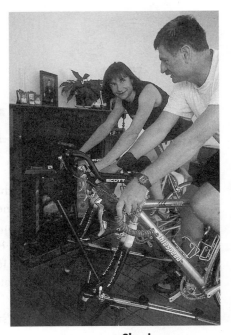

Sharing your spinning with a friend is fun and suits the intermediate athlete.

To summarise

USING THE PROGRAMME ON THE ROAD

You do the specified duration or distance given in the programme, and refer to the subtext number beside it and the explanation in the 'Spinning workouts' chapter for what to do *within* the workout. Use the workout examples immediately after the explanation for ideas on the types of training to do. Ignore the durations given in the workout examples.

USING THE PROGRAMME ON YOUR STATIONARY TRAINER

Refer to the programme and look up the subtext number for a particular training day (ignore the specified training volume). Look up the explanations in the 'Spinning workouts' chapter for a description of how to do the training and for workouts that you can use.

How hard do I go?

Transfer the training heart rates that you have already calculated (pages 41–43) to the heart rate column in the workouts; you will then have your own individual training intensities for all the varieties of training you will do in your programme.

Making sure the programme suits you

The programmes given are examples of how to achieve your training goals. If you want to write your own programme, consult *The Power to Perform*.

Discussing your training with a coach or an experienced athlete is very useful. Use the experience around you — it's hard to learn from your mistakes; it's easier to learn from someone else's.

Choosing your training level

The workouts (pages 82–146) have two different training levels (providing specific workout quantities). You will need to select the level that best suits you.

Intermediate sport

- You want to get the most out of your training on limited time.
- You are in your first year of the sport.
- You are relaxed about your training and competition (you want to be involved, not competitive).
- You are prepared to invest a moderate amount of time in the sport but there are other things in life.
- You're keen but having fun is more important than doing really well.
- You've been doing your sport for quite a while and are happy with your level of commitment.

Advanced sport

- You are serious.
- You are experienced (in the sport for 3–5 years).
- You want to do well.

Points to note before starting your programme

- Some people mistakenly think that the closer you follow a programme, the better the chances of top performance. This is in fact not true. Listen to your body first, then look at the programme, and then decide how you will train for the day or week.

- Without recovery there is no improvement. Without improvement there are no increases in performance. Recovery is very important.

- Do not try to keep your log-book numbers straight. Your programme is a plan, reality is different. You should miss around 10% of the programme.

- Never try to catch up a missed workout. If it's gone, it's gone. You will destroy the balance of your programme if you try to catch up.

- Cruise on your easy days so you can save up your energy for your harder (long, hills, speed) days. In Base, your long days have highest priority with hills being next: in Speed for longer distance events, long is still most important followed by speed, hills and finally easy. Speed phases for shorter distance events have speed as the highest priority, with hills next and finally long. Always think in your workouts, 'Am I going to be fresh enough for my next key session?' You may even cut your workout on an easy day to ensure you are ready for your high-priority session.

- Keep a log-book. Log-books ensure that you have a record of training. If your training went optimally, you have a record of how you did it. You can use this again with some refinements for your next build-up. This way you are learning what forms of training work and which are in-effective. This allows far greater improvements in training from one build-up to the next. Also, if you are having problems in training with increasing your performance, a log-book will act as a guide to discovering what your training errors are. This can then be rectified.

- Don't stick to your heart rates like 'glue' — they are designed to give you a general intensity or 'average' intensity. Try to spend most of your time at the training heart rates but not all the time. There is nothing wrong with your heart rate going up because you went up a hill or you raced someone for 5–15 minutes. If your training heart rates seem wrong, particularly if they are not calculated from a test, use a more advanced method for assessing heart rates.

- Be patient. While this programme will help your performance, it generally takes two to three build-ups to get things running smoothly.

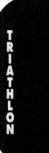

Race: Triathlon (sprint/Olympic)
Race date: 20 April
Training starts: 30 December

Maximum distance for the 100% week
Swim: 4 km
Bike: 100 kms
Run: 16 km

Mileage profile

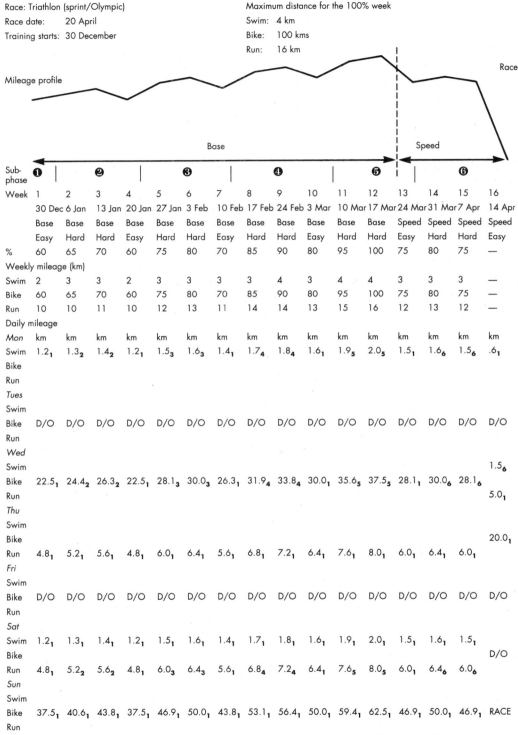

Sub-phase	❶			❷			❸			❹			❺		❻	
Week	1	2	3	4	5	6	7	8	9	10	11	12	13	14	15	16
	30 Dec	6 Jan	13 Jan	20 Jan	27 Jan	3 Feb	10 Feb	17 Feb	24 Feb	3 Mar	10 Mar	17 Mar	24 Mar	31 Mar	7 Apr	14 Apr
	Base	Base	Base	Base	Base	Base	Base	Base	Base	Base	Base	Base	Speed	Speed	Speed	Speed
	Easy	Hard	Hard	Easy	Hard	Hard	Easy	Hard	Hard	Easy	Hard	Hard	Easy	Hard	Hard	Easy
%	60	65	70	60	75	80	70	85	90	80	95	100	75	80	75	—
Weekly mileage (km)																
Swim	2	3	3	2	3	3	3	3	4	3	4	4	3	3	3	—
Bike	60	65	70	60	75	80	70	85	90	80	95	100	75	80	75	—
Run	10	10	11	10	12	13	11	14	14	13	15	16	12	13	12	—
Daily mileage																
Mon	km	km	km	km	km	km	km	km	km	km	km	km	km	km	km	km
Swim	1.2_1	1.3_2	1.4_2	1.2_1	1.5_3	1.6_3	1.4_1	1.7_4	1.8_4	1.6_1	1.9_5	2.0_5	1.5_1	1.6_6	1.5_6	$.6_1$
Bike																
Run																
Tues																
Swim																
Bike	D/O	D/O	D/O	D/O	D/O	D/O	D/O	D/O	D/O	D/O	D/O	D/O	D/O	D/O	D/O	D/O
Run																
Wed																
Swim																1.5_6
Bike	22.5_1	24.4_2	26.3_2	22.5_1	28.1_3	30.0_3	26.3_1	31.9_4	33.8_4	30.0_1	35.6_5	37.5_5	28.1_1	30.0_6	28.1_6	
Run																5.0_1
Thu																
Swim																
Bike																20.0_1
Run	4.8_1	5.2_1	5.6_1	4.8_1	6.0_1	6.4_1	5.6_1	6.8_1	7.2_1	6.4_1	7.6_1	8.0_1	6.0_1	6.4_1	6.0_1	
Fri																
Swim																
Bike	D/O	D/O	D/O	D/O	D/O	D/O	D/O	D/O	D/O	D/O	D/O	D/O	D/O	D/O	D/O	D/O
Run																
Sat																
Swim	1.2_1	1.3_1	1.4_1	1.2_1	1.5_1	1.6_1	1.4_1	1.7_1	1.8_1	1.6_1	1.9_1	2.0_1	1.5_1	1.6_1	1.5_1	
Bike																D/O
Run	4.8_1	5.2_2	5.6_2	4.8_1	6.0_3	6.4_3	5.6_1	6.8_4	7.2_4	6.4_1	7.6_5	8.0_5	6.0_1	6.4_6	6.0_6	
Sun																
Swim																
Bike	37.5_1	40.6_1	43.8_1	37.5_1	46.9_1	50.0_1	43.8_1	53.1_1	56.4_1	50.0_1	59.4_1	62.5_1	46.9_1	50.0_1	46.9_1	RACE
Run																

The bold subscript numerals refer to subphases; see chapter 2. Refer to *Precision Training* or *The Power to Perform* for swim/run training information.

Race: Triathlon (sprint/Olympic)
Race date: 20 April
Training starts: 30 December

Maximum distance for the 100% week
Swim: 4 km
Bike: 180 km
Run: 25 km

Mileage profile

Base   Speed

Sub-phase	❶	❷	❸	❹	❺	❻

Week	1	2	3	4	5	6	7	8	9	10	11	12	13	14	15	16
	30 Dec	6 Jan	13 Jan	20 Jan	27 Jan	3 Feb	10 Feb	17 Feb	24 Feb	3 Mar	10 Mar	17 Mar	24 Mar	31 Mar	7 Apr	14 Apr
	Base	Base	Base	Base	Base	Base	Base	Base	Base	Base	Base	Speed	Speed	Speed	Speed	Speed
	Easy	Hard	Hard	Easy	Hard	Hard	Easy	Hard	Hard	Easy	Hard	Hard	Easy	Hard	Hard	Easy
%	65	70	75	65	80	85	70	90	95	80	100	95	75	85	75	—
Weekly mileage (km)																
Swim	3	3	3	3	3	3	3	4	4	3	4	4	3	3	3	—
Bike	117	126	135	117	144	153	126	162	171	144	180	171	135	153	135	—
Run	16	18	19	16	20	21	18	23	24	20	25	24	19	21	19	—

Daily mileage

Mon	km	km	km	km	km	km	km	km	km	km	km	km	km	km	km	km
Swim	$.8_1$	$.8_1$	$.9_1$	$.8_1$	1.0_1	$.8_1$	1.1_1	1.1_1	1.0_1	1.2_1	1.1_1	$.9_1$	1.0_1	$.9_1$	1.5_1	
Bike																
Run	4.1_1	4.4_2	4.7_2	4.1_1	5.0_2	5.3_2	4.4_1	$5.6_{2\text{-}3}$	$5.9_{2\text{-}3}$	5.0_1	$6.3_{2\text{-}4}$	$5.9_{2\text{-}4}$	4.7_1	$5.3_{2\text{-}4}$	$4.7_{2\text{-}4}$	6.0_1
Tues																
Swim																
Bike	26.0_1	28.0_2	30.0_2	26.0_1	32.0_3	34.0_3	28.0_1	36.0_4	38.0_4	32.0_1	40.0_5	38.0_5	30.0_1	34.0_6	30.0_6	30.0_6
Run																
Wed																
Swim	$.8_1$	$.8_2$	$.9_2$	$.8_1$	1.0_2	1.0_2	$.8_1$	$1.12_{2\text{-}3}$	$1.1_{2\text{-}3}$	1.0_1	$1.2_{2\text{-}4}$	$1.1_{2\text{-}4}$	$.9_1$	$1.0_{2\text{-}4}$	$.9_{2\text{-}4}$	1.5_1
Bike																
Run	8.1_1	8.8_1	9.4_1	8.1_1	10.0_1	10.6_1	8.8_1	11.3_1	11.9_1	10.0_1	12.5_1	11.9_1	9.4_1	10.6_1	9.4_1	6.0_1
Thur																
Swim																
Bike	26.0_1	28.0_2	30.0_2	26.0_1	32.0_2	34.0_2	28.0_1	36.0_3	38.0_3	32.0_1	40.0_4	38.0_4	30.0_1	34.0_4	30.0_4	20.0_1
Run																
Fri																
Swim																
Bike	D/O	D/O	D/O	D/O	D/O	D/O	D/O	D/O	D/O	D/O	D/O	D/O	D/O	D/O	D/O	D/O
Run																
Sat																
Swim	1.0_1	1.1_2	1.2_2	1.0_1	1.3_5	1.4_3	1.1_1	1.4_4	1.5_4	1.3_1	1.6_5	1.5_5	1.2_1	$1.4_{5\text{-}6}$	$1.2_{5\text{-}6}$	
Bike																D/O
Run	4.1_1	4.4_2	4.7_2	4.1_1	5.0_3	5.3_3	4.4_1	5.6_4	5.9_4	5.0_1	6.3_5	5.9_5	4.7_1	$5.3_{5\text{-}6}$	$4.7_{5\text{-}6}$	
Sun																
Swim																
Bike	65.0_1	70.0_1	75.0_1	65.0_1	80.0_1	85.0_1	70.0_1	90.0_1	95.0_1	80.0_1	100.0_1	95.0_1	75.0_1	85.0_1	75.0_1	RACE
Run																

Base 1 would occur first. **The bold subscript numerals refer to subphases; see chapter 2. Refer to *Precision Training* or *The Power to Perform* for swim/run training information.**

Race: Triathlon (Olympic/half-Ironman)
Race date: 20 April
Training starts: 30 December

Maximum distance for the 100% week
Swim: 12 km
Bike: 240 km
Run: 50 km

Mileage profile

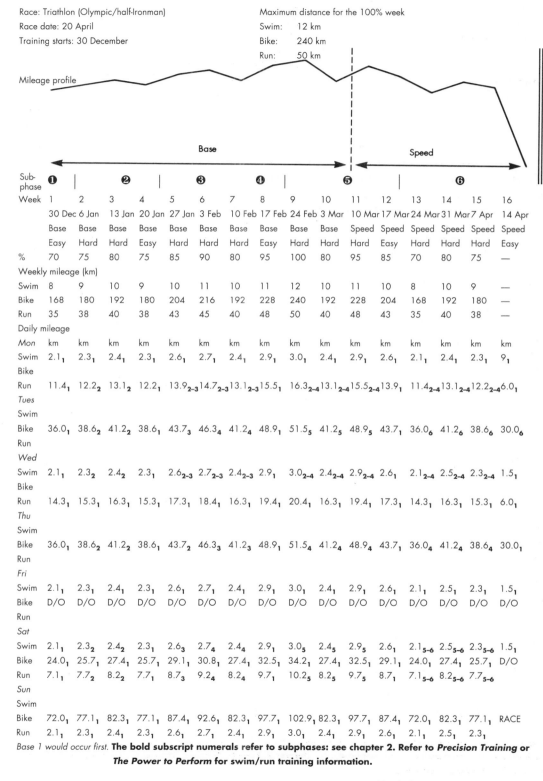

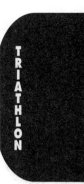

Sub-phase	❶		❷		❸		❹		❺			❻				
Phase	Base										Speed					
Week	1	2	3	4	5	6	7	8	9	10	11	12	13	14	15	16
	30 Dec	6 Jan	13 Jan	20 Jan	27 Jan	3 Feb	10 Feb	17 Feb	24 Feb	3 Mar	10 Mar	17 Mar	24 Mar	31 Mar	7 Apr	14 Apr
	Base	Base	Base	Base	Base	Base	Base	Base	Base	Base	Speed	Speed	Speed	Speed	Speed	Speed
	Easy	Hard	Hard	Easy	Hard	Hard	Hard	Easy	Hard	Hard	Hard	Easy	Hard	Hard	Hard	Easy
%	70	75	80	75	85	90	80	95	100	80	95	85	70	80	75	—
Weekly mileage (km)																
Swim	8	9	10	9	10	11	10	11	12	10	11	10	8	10	9	—
Bike	168	180	192	180	204	216	192	228	240	192	228	204	168	192	180	—
Run	35	38	40	38	43	45	40	48	50	40	48	43	35	40	38	—
Daily mileage																
Mon	km	km	km	km	km	km	km	km	km	km	km	km	km	km	km	km
Swim	2.1_1	2.3_1	2.4_1	2.3_1	2.6_1	2.7_1	2.4_1	2.9_1	3.0_1	2.4_1	2.9_1	2.6_1	2.1_1	2.4_1	2.3_1	9_1
Bike																
Run	11.4_1	12.2_2	13.1_2	12.2_1	13.9_{2-3}	14.7_{2-3}	13.1_{2-3}	15.5_1	16.3_{2-4}	13.1_{2-4}	15.5_{2-4}	13.9_1	11.4_{2-4}	13.1_{2-4}	12.2_{2-4}	6.0_1
Tues																
Swim																
Bike	36.0_1	38.6_2	41.2_2	38.6_1	43.7_3	46.3_4	41.2_4	48.9_1	51.5_5	41.2_5	48.9_5	43.7_1	36.0_6	41.2_6	38.6_6	30.0_6
Run																
Wed																
Swim	2.1_1	2.3_2	2.4_2	2.3_1	2.6_{2-3}	2.7_{2-3}	2.4_{2-3}	2.9_1	3.0_{2-4}	2.4_{2-4}	2.9_{2-4}	2.6_1	2.1_{2-4}	2.5_{2-4}	2.3_{2-4}	1.5_1
Bike																
Run	14.3_1	15.3_1	16.3_1	15.3_1	17.3_1	18.4_1	16.3_1	19.4_1	20.4_1	16.3_1	19.4_1	17.3_1	14.3_1	16.3_1	15.3_1	6.0_1
Thu																
Swim																
Bike	36.0_1	38.6_2	41.2_2	38.6_1	43.7_2	46.3_3	41.2_3	48.9_1	51.5_4	41.2_4	48.9_4	43.7_1	36.0_4	41.2_4	38.6_4	30.0_1
Run																
Fri																
Swim	2.1_1	2.3_1	2.4_1	2.3_1	2.6_1	2.7_1	2.4_1	2.9_1	3.0_1	2.4_1	2.9_1	2.6_1	2.1_1	2.5_1	2.3_1	1.5_1
Bike	D/O	D/O	D/O	D/O	D/O	D/O	D/O	D/O	D/O	D/O	D/O	D/O	D/O	D/O	D/O	D/O
Run																
Sat																
Swim	2.1_1	2.3_2	2.4_2	2.3_1	2.6_3	2.7_4	2.4_4	2.9_1	3.0_5	2.4_5	2.9_5	2.6_1	2.1_{5-6}	2.5_{5-6}	2.3_{5-6}	1.5_1
Bike	24.0_1	25.7_1	27.4_1	25.7_1	29.1_1	30.8_1	27.4_1	32.5_1	34.2_1	27.4_1	32.5_1	29.1_1	24.0_1	27.4_1	25.7_1	D/O
Run	7.1_1	7.7_2	8.2_2	7.7_1	8.7_3	9.2_4	8.2_4	9.7_1	10.2_5	8.2_5	9.7_5	8.7_1	7.1_{5-6}	8.2_{5-6}	7.7_{5-6}	
Sun																
Swim																
Bike	72.0_1	77.1_1	82.3_1	77.1_1	87.4_1	92.6_1	82.3_1	97.7_1	102.9_1	82.3_1	97.7_1	87.4_1	72.0_1	82.3_1	77.1_1	RACE
Run	2.1_1	2.3_1	2.4_1	2.3_1	2.6_1	2.7_1	2.4_1	2.9_1	3.0_1	2.4_1	2.9_1	2.6_1	2.1_1	2.5_1	2.3_1	

Base 1 would occur first. **The bold subscript numerals refer to subphases: see chapter 2. Refer to** *Precision Training* **or** *The Power to Perform* **for swim/run training information.**

Race: Ironman
Race date: 20 April
Training starts: 30 December

Maximum distance for the 100% week
Swim: 9 km
Bike: 280 km
Run: 60 km

Mileage profile

Base — Speed

Sub-phase	❶		❷		❸		❹		❺		❻					
Week	1	2	3	4	5	6	7	8	9	10	11	12	13	14	15	16
	30 Dec	6 Jan	13 Jan	20 Jan	27 Jan	3 Feb	10 Feb	17 Feb	24 Feb	3 Mar	10 Mar	17 Mar	24 Mar	31 Mar	7 Apr	14 Apr
	Base	Base	Base	Base	Base	Base	Base	Base	Base	Base	Speed	Speed	Speed	Speed	Speed	Speed
	Easy	Hard	Hard	Easy	Hard	Hard	Easy	Hard	Hard	Easy	Hard	Hard	Easy	Hard	Hard	Easy
%	58	72	79	65	86	93	72	93	100	79	93	100	72	86	72	—

Weekly mileage (km)

	1	2	3	4	5	6	7	8	9	10	11	12	13	14	15	16
Swim	5	6	7	6	8	8	6	8	9	7	8	9	6	8	6	—
Bike	162	202	221	182	241	260	202	260	280	221	260	280	202	241	172	—
Run	35	43	47	39	52	56	43	56	60	47	56	60	43	52	43	—

Daily mileage

Mon (km)

	1	2	3	4	5	6	7	8	9	10	11	12	13	14	15	16
Swim	1.6_1	1.9_1	2.1_1	1.8_1	2.3_1	2.5_1	1.9_1	2.5_1	2.7_1	2.1_1	2.5_1	2.7_1	1.9_1	2.3_1	1.9_1	$.8_1$
Bike																
Run	10.5_1	13.1_2	14.4_2	11.8_1	15.6_2	16.9_2	13.1_1	$16.9_{2\text{-}3}$	$18.2_{2\text{-}3}$	14.4_1	$16.9_{2\text{-}4}$	$18.2_{2\text{-}4}$	13.1_1	$15.6_{2\text{-}4}$	$13.1_{2\text{-}4}$	6.0_1

Tues

	1	2	3	4	5	6	7	8	9	10	11	12	13	14	15	16
Swim																
Bike	34.8_1	43.2_2	47.4_2	39.0_1	51.6_3	55.8_3	43.2_1	55.8_4	60.0_4	47.4_1	55.8_5	60.0_5	43.2_1	51.6_6	43.2_6	30.0_6
Run																

Wed

	1	2	3	4	5	6	7	8	9	10	11	12	13	14	15	16
Swim	1.6_1	1.9_2	2.1_2	1.8_1	2.3_2	2.5_2	1.9_1	$2.5_{2\text{-}3}$	$2.7_{2\text{-}3}$	2.1_1	$2.5_{2\text{-}4}$	$2.7_{2\text{-}4}$	1.9_1	$2.3_{2\text{-}4}$	$1.9_{2\text{-}4}$	1.5_1
Bike																
Run	15.8_1	19.6_1	21.5_1	17.7_1	23.5_1	25.4_1	19.6_1	25.4_1	27.3_1	21.5_1	25.4_1	27.3_1	19.6_1	23.5_1	19.6_1	6.0_1

Thu

	1	2	3	4	5	6	7	8	9	10	11	12	13	14	15	16
Swim																
Bike	23.2_1	28.8_2	31.6_2	26.0_1	34.4_2	37.2_2	28.8_1	37.2_3	40.0_3	31.6_1	37.2_4	40.0_4	28.8_1	34.4_4	28.8_4	20.0_1
Run																

Fri

	1	2	3	4	5	6	7	8	9	10	11	12	13	14	15	16
Swim																
Bike	D/O	D/O	D/O	D/O	D/O	D/O	D/O	D/O	D/O	D/O	D/O	D/O	D/O	D/O	D/O	D/O
Run																

Sat

	1	2	3	4	5	6	7	8	9	10	11	12	13	14	15	16
Swim	2.1_1	2.6_2	2.8_2	2.3_1	3.1_3	3.3_3	2.6_1	3.3_4	3.6_4	2.8_1	3.3_5	3.6_5	2.6_1	$3.1_{5\text{-}6}$	$2.6_{5\text{-}6}$	
Bike																D/O
Run	8.4_1	10.5_2	11.5_2	9.5_1	12.5_3	13.5_3	10.5_1	13.5_4	14.5_4	11.5_1	13.5_5	14.5_5	10.5_1	$12.5_{5\text{-}6}$	$10.5_{5\text{-}6}$	

Sun

	1	2	3	4	5	6	7	8	9	10	11	12	13	14	15	16
Swim																
Bike	104.4_1	129.6_1	142.2_1	117.0_1	154.8_1	167.4_1	129.6_1	167.4_1	180.0_1	142.2_1	167.4_1	180.0_1	129.6_1	154.8_1	100.0_1	RACE
Run																

Note: mileages would be set based on this guide. In Ironman training more 180 km bike rides may be trained. Base 1 would occur first.
The bold subscript numerals refer to subphases; see chapter 2. Refer to *Precision Training* or *The Power to Perform* for swim/run training information.

TRIATHLON

Race: Ironman
Race date: 20 April
Training starts: 30 December

Maximum distance for the 100% week
Swim: 12 km
Bike: 360 km
Run: 75 km

Mileage profile

Base

Speed

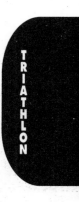
Sub-phase ❶ ❷ ❸ ❹ ❺ ❻

Week	1	2	3	4	5	6	7	8	9	10	11	12	13	14	15	16
	30 Dec	6 Jan	13 Jan	20 Jan	27 Jan	3 Feb	10 Feb	17 Feb	24 Feb	3 Mar	10 Mar	17 Mar	24 Mar	31 Mar	7 Apr	14 Apr
	Base	Base	Base	Base	Base	Base	Base	Base	Speed	Speed	Speed	Speed	Speed	Speed	Speed	Speed
	Easy	Hard	Hard	Hard	Hard	Easy	Hard	Hard	Hard	Hard	Easy	Hard	Hard	Hard	Hard	Easy
%	58	65	72	79	86	65	93	100	93	100	72	93	100	72	65	—
Weekly mileage (km)																
Swim	7	8	9	9	10	8	11	12	11	12	9	11	12	9	8	—
Bike	209	234	259	284	310	234	335	360	335	360	259	335	360	259	217	—
Run	44	49	54	59	65	49	70	75	70	75	54	70	75	54	49	—

Daily mileage

Mon	km	km	km	km	km	km	km	km	km	km	km	km	km	km	km	km
Swim	1.7$_1$	2.0$_1$	2.2$_1$	2.4$_1$	2.6$_1$	2.0$_1$	2.8$_1$	3.0$_1$	2.8$_1$	3.0$_1$	2.2$_1$	2.8$_1$	3.0$_1$	2.2$_1$	2.0$_1$	.9$_1$
Bike																
Run	11.6$_1$	13.0$_2$	14.4$_2$	15.8$_{2-3}$	17.2$_{2-3}$	13.0$_1$	18.6$_{2-3}$	20.0$_{2-3}$	18.6$_{2-4}$	20.0$_{2-4}$	14.4$_1$	18.6$_{2-4}$	20.0$_{2-4}$	14.4$_{2-4}$	13.0$_{2-4}$	10.0$_1$
Tues																
Swim																
Bike	32.0$_1$	35.9$_2$	39.7$_2$	43.6$_3$	47.5$_3$	35.9$_1$	51.3$_4$	55.2$_4$	51.3$_5$	55.2$_5$	39.7$_1$	51.3$_6$	55.2$_6$	39.7$_6$	35.9$_6$	30.0$_6$
Run																
Wed																
Swim	1.7$_1$	2.0$_2$	2.2$_2$	2.4$_{2-3}$	2.6$_{2-3}$	2.0$_1$	2.8$_{2-3}$	3.0$_{2-3}$	2.8$_{2-4}$	3.0$_{2-4}$	2.2$_1$	2.8$_{2-4}$	3.0$_{2-4}$	2.2$_{2-4}$	2.0$_{2-4}$	2.0$_1$
Bike																
Run	20.9$_1$	23.4$_1$	25.9$_1$	28.4$_1$	31.0$_1$	23.4$_1$	33.5$_1$	36.0$_1$	33.5$_1$	36.0$_1$	25.9$_1$	33.5$_1$	36.0$_1$	25.9$_1$	23.4$_1$	10.0$_1$
Thur																
Swim																
Bike	37.6$_1$	42.1$_1$	46.7$_1$	51.2$_2$	55.7$_2$	42.1$_1$	60.3$_3$	64.8$_3$	60.3$_4$	64.8$_4$	46.7$_1$	60.3$_4$	64.8$_4$	46.7$_4$	42.1$_4$	30.0$_1$
Run																
Fri																
Swim	1.7$_1$	2.0$_1$	2.2$_1$	2.4$_1$	2.6$_1$	2.0$_1$	2.8$_1$	3.0$_1$	2.8$_1$	3.0$_1$	2.2$_1$	2.8$_1$	3.0$_1$	2.2$_1$	2.0$_1$	.9$_1$
Bike																
Run																
Sat																
Swim	1.7$_1$	2.0$_2$	2.2$_2$	2.4$_3$	2.6$_3$	2.0$_1$	2.8$_4$	3.0$_4$	2.8$_5$	3.0$_5$	2.2$_1$	2.8$_{5-6}$	3.0$_{5-6}$	2.2$_{5-6}$	2.0$_{5-6}$	
Bike	34.8$_1$	39.0$_1$	43.2$_1$	47.4$_1$	51.6$_1$	39.0$_1$	55.8$_1$	60.0$_1$	55.8$_1$	60.0$_1$	43.2$_1$	55.8$_1$	60.0$_1$	43.2$_1$	39.0$_1$	D/O
Run	9.3$_1$	10.4$_2$	11.5$_2$	12.6$_3$	13.8$_3$	10.4$_1$	14.9$_4$	16.0$_4$	14.9$_5$	16.0$_5$	11.5$_1$	14.9$_{5-6}$	16.0$_{5-6}$	11.5$_{5-6}$	10.4$_{5-6}$	
Sun																
Swim																
Bike	104.4$_1$	117.0$_1$	129.6$_1$	142.2$_1$	134.8$_1$	117.0$_1$	167.4$_1$	180.0$_1$	167.4$_1$	180.0$_1$	129.6$_1$	167.4$_1$	180.0$_1$	129.6$_1$	100.0$_1$	RACE
Run	1.7$_1$	2.0$_1$	2.2$_1$	2.4$_1$	2.6$_1$	2.0$_1$	2.8$_1$	3.0$_1$	2.8$_1$	3.0$_1$	2.2$_1$	2.8$_1$	3.0$_1$	2.2$_1$	2.0$_1$	

Note: mileages would be set based on this guide. In Ironman training more 180 km bike rides may be trained. Base 1 would occur first.

The bold subscript numerals refer to subphases; see chapter 2. Refer to *Precision Training* or *The Power to Perform* for swim/run training information.

Race: Duathlon 4 km/20/ km/ 4 km
Race date: 20 April
Training starts: 30 December

Maximum distance for the 100% week
Run: 38 km
Bike: 160 km

Mileage profile

	Base										Speed					
Sub-phase	❶		❷		❸		❹				❺		❻			
Week	1	2	3	4	5	6	7	8	9	10	11	12	13	14	15	16
	30 Dec	6 Jan	13 Jan	20 Jan	27 Jan	3 Feb	10 Feb	17 Feb	24 Feb	3 Mar	10 Mar	17 Mar	24 Mar	31 Mar	7 Apr	14 Apr
	Base	Base	Base	Base	Base	Base	Base	Base	Base	Base	Speed	Speed	Speed	Speed	Speed	Speed
	Easy	Hard	Hard	Easy	Hard	Hard	Hard	Easy	Hard	Hard	Hard	Easy	Hard	Hard	Hard	Easy
%	51	58	65	58	72	79	86	72	93	100	93	72	86	79	65	—
Weekly mileage (km)																
Run	19	22	25	22	27	30	33	27	35	38	35	27	33	30	25	—
Bike	82	93	104	93	115	126	138	115	149	160	149	115	138	126	104	—
Daily mileage																
Mon	km	km	km	km	km	km	km	km	km	km	km	km	km	km	km	km
Run	5.1_1	5.8_2	6.5_2	5.8_1	7.2_2	7.9_2	$8.6_{2\text{-}3}$	7.2_1	$9.3_{2\text{-}4}$	$10.0_{2\text{-}4}$	$9.3_{2\text{-}4}$	7.2_1	$8.6_{2\text{-}4}$	$7.9_{2\text{-}4}$	$6.5_{2\text{-}4}$	6.0_1
Bike																
Tues																
Run																
Bike	20.4_1	23.2_2	26_2	23.2_1	28.8_3	31.6_3	34.4_4	28.8_1	37.2_5	40.0_5	37.2_5	28.8_1	34.4_6	31.6_6	26_6	20.0_6
Wed																
Run	9.2_1	10.4_1	11.7_1	10.4_1	13.0_1	14.2_1	15.5_1	15.0_1	16.7_1	18.0_1	16.7_1	13.0_1	15.5_1	14.2_1	11.7_1	6.0_1
Bike																
Thur																
Run																
Bike	20.4_1	23.2_2	26_2	23.2_1	28.8_2	21.6_2	34.4_3	28.8_1	37.2_4	40.0_4	37.2_4	28.8_1	34.4_4	31.6_4	26_4	20.0_1
Fri																
Run	D/O	D/O	D/O	D/O	D/O	D/O	D/O	D/O	D/O	D/O	D/O	D/O	D/O	D/O	D/O	D/O
Bike																
Sat																
Run	4.1_1	4.6_2	5.2_2	4.6_1	5.8_3	6.3_3	6.9_4	5.8_1	7.4_5	8.0_5	$2\times3.7_5$	$2\times2.9_1$	$2\times3.4_{5\text{-}6}$	$2\times3.2_{5\text{-}6}$	$2\times2.0_{5\text{-}6}$	D/O
Bike	10.2_1	11.6_1	13.0_1	11.6_1	14.4_1	15.8_1	17.2_1	14.4_1	18.6_1	20.0_1	18.6_1	14.4_1	17.2_1	15.8_1	13_1	
Sun																
Run	1.0_1	1.2_1	1.3_1	1.2_1	1.4_1	1.6_1	1.7_1	1.4_1	1.9_1	2.0_1	1.9_1	1.4_1	1.7_1	1.6_1	1.3_1	RACE
Bike	30.6_1	34.8_1	39.0_1	34.8_1	43.2_1	47.4_1	51.6_1	43.2_1	55.8_1	60.0_1	55.8_1	43.2_1	51.6_1	47.4_1	39.0_1	

The bold subscript numerals refer to subphases; see chapter 2. Refer to *Precision Training* or *The Power to Perform* for training information.

Race: Powerman 10 km/60 km/10 km
Race date: 20 April
Training starts: 30 December

Maximum distance for the 100% week
Run: 69 km
Bike: 320 km

Mileage profile

Sub-phase	❶		❷		❸		❹		❺		❻					
						Base							Speed			
Week	1	2	3	4	5	6	7	8	9	10	11	12	13	14	15	16
	30 Dec	6 Jan	13 Jan	20 Jan	27 Jan	3 Feb	10 Feb	17 Feb	24 Feb	3 Mar	10 Mar	17 Mar	24 Mar	31 Mar	7 Apr	14 Apr
	Base	Base	Base	Base	Base	Base	Base	Base	Base	Base	Speed	Speed	Speed	Speed	Speed	Speed
	Easy	Hard	Hard	Easy	Hard	Hard	Hard	Easy	Hard	Hard	Hard	Easy	Hard	Hard	Hard	Easy
%	51	58	65	58	72	79	86	72	93	100	93	72	86	79	65	—

Weekly mileage (km)

	1	2	3	4	5	6	7	8	9	10	11	12	13	14	15	16
Run	36	40	45	40	50	55	59	50	64	69	64	50	59	55	45	—
Bike	163	186	208	186	230	253	275	230	298	320	298	230	275	253	208	—

Daily mileage

Mon	km	km	km	km	km	km	km	km	km	km	km	km	km	km	km	km
Run	7.7$_1$	8.7$_2$	9.8$_2$	8.7$_1$	10.8$_2$	11.9$_2$	12.9$_{2-3}$	10.8$_1$	14.0$_{2-4}$	15.0$_{2-4}$	14.0$_{2-4}$	10.8$_1$	12.9$_{2-4}$	11.9$_{2-4}$	9.8$_{2-4}$	6.0$_1$
Bike																
Tues																
Run																
Bike	30.6$_1$	34.8$_2$	39.0$_2$	34.8$_1$	43.2$_3$	47.4$_3$	51.6$_4$	43.2$_1$	55.8$_5$	60.0$_5$	55.8$_5$	43.2$_1$	51.6$_6$	47.4$_6$	39.0$_6$	30.0$_6$
Wed																
Run	12.8$_1$	14.5$_1$	16.3$_1$	14.5$_1$	18.0$_1$	19.8$_1$	21.5$_1$	18.0$_1$	23.3$_1$	25$_1$	23.3$_1$	18.0$_1$	21.5$_1$	19.8$_1$	16.3$_1$	6.0$_1$
Bike	15.3$_1$	17.4$_1$	19.5$_1$	17.4$_1$	21.6$_1$	23.7$_1$	25.8$_1$	21.6$_1$	27.9$_1$	30.0$_1$	27.9$_1$	21.6$_1$	25.8$_1$	23.7$_1$	19.5$_1$	20.0$_1$
Thur																
Run	3.1$_1$	3.5$_1$	3.9$_1$	3.5$_1$	4.3$_1$	4.7$_1$	5.2$_1$	4.3$_1$	5.6$_1$	6.0$_1$	5.6$_1$	4.3$_1$	5.2$_1$	4.7$_1$	3.9$_1$	5.0$_1$
Bike	25.5$_1$	29.0$_2$	32.5$_2$	29.0$_1$	36.0$_2$	39.5$_2$	43.0$_3$	36.0$_1$	46.5$_4$	50.0$_4$	46.5$_4$	36.0$_1$	43.0$_4$	39.5$_4$	32.5$_4$	30.0$_1$
Fri																
Run	D/O	D/O	D/O	D/O	D/O	D/O	D/O	D/O	D/O	D/O	D/O	D/O	D/O	D/O	D/O	D/O
Bike																
Sat																
Run	10.2$_1$	11.6$_2$	13.0$_2$	11.6$_1$	14.4$_3$	15.8$_3$	17.2$_4$	14.4$_1$	18.6$_5$	20.0$_5$	2×9.3$_5$	2×7.2$_1$	2×8.6$_{5-6}$	2×7.9$_{5-6}$	2×6.5$_{5-6}$	D/O
Bike	30.6$_1$	34.8$_2$	39.0$_1$	34.8$_1$	43.2$_1$	47.4$_1$	51.6$_1$	43.2$_1$	55.8$_1$	60.0$_1$	55.8$_1$	43.2$_1$	51.6$_1$	47.4$_1$	39.0$_1$	
Sun																
Run	1.5$_1$	1.7$_1$	2.0$_1$	1.7$_1$	2.2$_1$	2.4$_1$	2.6$_1$	2.2$_1$	2.8$_1$	3.0$_1$	2.8$_1$	2.2$_1$	2.6$_1$	2.4$_1$	2.0$_1$	RACE
Bike	61.2$_1$	69.6$_1$	78.0$_1$	69.6$_1$	86.4$_1$	94.8$_1$	103.2$_1$	86.4$_1$	111.6$_1$	120.0$_1$	111.6$_1$	86.4$_1$	103.2$_1$	94.8$_1$	78.0$_1$	

The bold subscript numerals refer to subphases; see chapter 2. Refer to *Precision Training* or *The Power to Perform* for training information.

To adjust from standard Powerman distances to Zolfingen Powerman distances, use the Ironman programmes on pages 68–9.

Race: Coast to Coast
Day 1: 2.8 km run/ 58 km cycle/26 km mountain run
Day 2: 15 km cycle/67 km kayak/70 km cycle
Race date: 20 April
Training starts: 30 December

Maximum distance for the 100% week
Cycle: 240 km
Run: 350 min
Kayak: 480 min

Mileage profile

Base — Speed

Sub-phase	❶		❷		❸		❹		❺		❻					
Week	1	2	3	4	5	6	7	8	9	10	11	12	13	14	15	16
	30 Dec	6 Jan	13 Jan	20 Jan	27 Jan	3 Feb	10 Feb	17 Feb	24 Feb	3 Mar	10 Mar	17 Mar	24 Mar	31 Mar	7 Apr	14 Apr
	Base Easy	Base Hard	Base Hard	Base Easy	Base Hard	Base Hard	Base Hard	Base Easy	Base Hard	Base Hard	Speed Hard	Speed Easy	Speed Hard	Speed Hard	Speed Hard	Speed Easy
%	51	58	65	58	72	79	86	72	93	100	93	72	100	79	65	—
Weekly mileage (km/min)																
Cycle	122	139	156	139	173	190	206	173	223	240	223	173	240	190	156	—
Run	179	203	228	203	252	277	301	252	325	350	325	252	350	277	228	—
Kayak	245	278	312	278	346	379	413	346	446	480	446	367	480	379	312	—
Daily mileage (km/min)																
Mon																
Cycle	20_1	23_2	26_2	23_1	29_3	32_3	34_3	29_1	37_4	40_4	37_5	29_1	40_6	32_6	26_6	40_6
Run	92_1	104_1	117_1	104_1	130_1	142_1	155_1	130_1	167_1	180_1	167_1	130_1	180_1	142_1	117_1	
Kayak																
Tues																
Cycle	31_1	35_2	39_2	35_1	43_2	47_2	52_2	43_1	56_3	60_3	37_4	29_1	40_4	32_4	26_4	
Run																
Kayak	31_1	35_1	39_1	35_1	43_1	47_1	52_1	43_1	56_1	60_1	84_1	65_1	90_1	71_1	59_1	30
Wed																
Cycle																
Run	46_1	52_2	59_2	52_1	65_3	71_3	77_3	65_1	84_4	90_4	84_5	65_1	$90_{5\text{–}6}$	$71_{5\text{–}6}$	$59_{5\text{–}6}$	20
Kayak	61_1	70_2	78_2	70_1	86_2	95_2	103_2	86_1	$112_{2\text{–}3}$	$120_{2\text{–}3}$	$112_{2\text{–}4}$	86_1	$120_{2\text{–}4}$	$95_{2\text{–}4}$	$78_{2\text{–}4}$	20
Thu																
Cycle	51_1	58_1	65_1	58_1	72_1	79_1	86_1	72_1	93_1	100_1	93_1	72_1	100_1	79_1	65_1	
Run	10_1	12_1	13_1	12_1	14_1	16_1	17_1	14_1	19_1	20_1	19_1	14_1	20_1	16_1	13_1	D/O
Kayak																
Fri	D/O	D/O	D/O	D/O	D/O	D/O	D/O	D/O	D/O	D/O	D/O	D/O	D/O	D/O	D/O	D/O
Sat																
Cycle	20_1	23_1	26_1	23_1	29_1	32_1	34_1	29_1	37_1	40_1	56_1	43_1	60_1	47_1	39_1	
Run	31_1	35_2	39_2	35_1	43_2	47_2	52_2	43_1	$56_{2\text{–}3}$	$60_{2\text{–}3}$	$56_{2\text{–}4}$	43_1	$60_{2\text{–}4}$	$47_{2\text{–}4}$	$39_{2\text{–}4}$	RACE
Kayak	31_1	35_2	39_2	35_1	43_3	47_3	52_3	43_1	56_4	60_4	56_5	43_1	$60_{5\text{–}6}$	$47_{5\text{–}6}$	$39_{5\text{–}6}$	
Sun																
Cycle																
Run																RACE
Kayak	122_1	139_1	156_1	139_1	173_1	190_1	206_1	173_1	223_1	240_1	223_1	173_1	240_1	190_1	156_1	

Base 1 would occur first. **The bold subscript numerals refer to subphases; see chapter 2. Refer to *Precision Training* or *The Power to Perform* for run/kayak training information.**

Cycle volumes are displayed in kilometres; kayak and running volumes are in minutes.

'Longest day' is the 1-day version of the original Coast to Coast. Training volumes need not alter much (up 5–10% if you're keen), but longer multidiscipline workouts would be needed (in the 3rd and 5th, or 3rd, 5th and 7th weeks back from the race).

Race: Mountains to sea
Day 1: 23 km run/ 61 km cycle/35 km kayak
Day 2: 87 kayak
Day 3: 30 km run/34 km cycle
Race date: 20 April
Training starts: 30 December

Maximum distance for the 100% week
Cycle: 190 km
Run: 420 min
Kayak: 540 min

Mileage profile

	Base										Speed					
Sub-phase	❶		❷		❸			❹		❺		❻				
Week	1	2	3	4	5	6	7	8	9	10	11	12	13	14	15	16
	30 Dec	6 Jan	13 Jan	20 Jan	27 Jan	3 Feb	10 Feb	17 Feb	24 Feb	3 Mar	10 Mar	17 Mar	24 Mar	31 Mar	7 Apr	14 Apr
	Base	Base	Base	Base	Base	Base	Base	Base	Base	Base	Speed	Speed	Speed	Speed	Speed	Speed
	Easy	Hard	Hard	Easy	Hard	Hard	Hard	Easy	Hard	Hard	Hard	Easy	Hard	Hard	Hard	Easy
%	51	58	65	58	72	79	86	72	93	100	93	72	100	79	65	—
Weekly mileage (km/min)																
Cycle	97	100	124	110	137	150	163	137	177	190	177	137	190	150	124	—
Run	214	244	273	244	302	332	361	302	391	420	391	288	420	332	273	—
Kayak	275	313	351	313	389	427	464	389	502	540	502	410	540	427	351	—
Daily mileage (km/min)																
Mon																
Cycle	20_1	23_2	26_2	23_1	29_3	32_3	34_3	29_1	37_4	40_4	37_5	29_1	40_6	32_6	26_6	
Run	92_1	104_1	117_1	104_1	130_1	142_1	155_1	130_1	167_1	180_1	167_1	130_1	180_1	142_1	117_1	30_1
Kayak																
Tues																
Cycle	20_1	23_2	26_2	23_1	29_2	32_2	34_2	29_1	37_3	40_3	28_4	22_1	30_4	24_4	20_4	30_1
Run																
Kayak	31_1	35_1	39_1	35_1	43_1	47_1	52_1	43_1	56_1	60_1	84_1	65_1	90_1	71_1	59_1	
Wed																
Cycle																
Run	46_1	52_2	59_2	52_1	65_3	71_3	77_3	65_1	84_4	90_4	85_5	65_1	$90_{5\text{-}6}$	$71_{5\text{-}6}$	$59_{5\text{-}6}$	30_1
Kayak	61_1	70_2	78_2	70_1	86_2	95_2	103_2	86_1	$112_{2\text{-}3}$	$120_{2\text{-}3}$	$112_{2\text{-}4}$	86_1	$120_{2\text{-}4}$	$95_{2\text{-}4}$	$78_{2\text{-}4}$	20_1
Thu																
Cycle	41_1	46_1	52_1	46_1	58_1	63_1	69_1	58_1	74_1	80_1	74_1	58_1	80_1	63_1	52_1	
Run	31_1	35_1	39_1	35_1	43_1	47_1	52_1	43_1	56_1	60_1	37_1	29_1	40_1	32_1	26_1	D/O
Fri	D/O	D/O	D/O	D/O	D/O	D/O	D/O	D/O	D/O	D/O	D/O	D/O	D/O	D/O	D/O	D/O
Sat																
Cycle	15_1	17_1	20_1	17_1	22_1	24_1	26_1	22_1	28_1	30_1	37_1	29_1	40_1	32_1	26_1	
Run	46_1	52_2	59_2	52_1	65_2	71_2	77_2	65_1	$84_{2\text{-}3}$	$90_{2\text{-}3}$	$84_{2\text{-}4}$	65_1	$90_{2\text{-}4}$	$71_{2\text{-}4}$	$59_{2\text{-}4}$	RACE
Kayak	31_1	35_2	39_2	35_1	43_3	47_3	52_3	43_1	56_4	60_4	56_5	43_1	$60_{5\text{-}6}$	$47_{5\text{-}6}$	$39_{5\text{-}6}$	
Sun																
Cycle																
Run																
Kayak	153_1	174_1	195_1	174_1	216_1	237_1	258_1	216_1	279_1	300_1	279_1	216_1	300_1	237_1	195_1	RACE

Base 1 would occur first.

Cycle volumes are displayed in kilometres; kayak and running volumes are in minutes.

The bold subscript numerals refer to subphases; see chapter 2. Refer to *Precision Training* or *The Power to Perform* for run/kayak training information.

Race: Cycle (40 km)
Race date: 20 April
Training starts: 30 December

Maximum distance for the 100% week
Cycle: 160 km

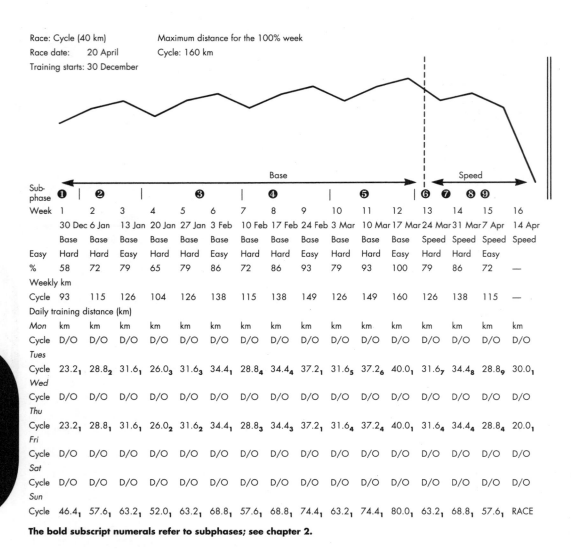

Sub-phase	❶	❷		❸		❹		❺		❻	❼	❽ ❾	
Week	1	2	3	4	5	6	7	8	9	10	11	12	13	14	15	16

Week	1	2	3	4	5	6	7	8	9	10	11	12	13	14	15	16
	30 Dec	6 Jan	13 Jan	20 Jan	27 Jan	3 Feb	10 Feb	17 Feb	24 Feb	3 Mar	10 Mar	17 Mar	24 Mar	31 Mar	7 Apr	14 Apr
	Base	Base	Base	Base	Base	Base	Base	Base	Base	Base	Base	Base	Speed	Speed	Speed	Speed
Easy	Hard	Hard	Easy	Hard	Hard	Easy	Hard	Hard	Easy	Hard	Hard	Easy	Hard	Hard	Easy	
%	58	72	79	65	79	86	72	86	93	79	93	100	79	86	72	—
Weekly km																
Cycle	93	115	126	104	126	138	115	138	149	126	149	160	126	138	115	—
Daily training distance (km)																
Mon	km	km	km	km	km	km	km	km	km	km	km	km	km	km	km	km
Cycle	D/O	D/O	D/O	D/O	D/O	D/O	D/O	D/O	D/O	D/O	D/O	D/O	D/O	D/O	D/O	D/O
Tues																
Cycle	23.2_1	28.8_2	31.6_1	26.0_3	31.6_3	34.4_1	28.8_4	34.4_4	37.2_1	31.6_5	37.2_6	40.0_1	31.6_7	34.4_8	28.8_9	30.0_1
Wed																
Cycle	D/O	D/O	D/O	D/O	D/O	D/O	D/O	D/O	D/O	D/O	D/O	D/O	D/O	D/O	D/O	D/O
Thu																
Cycle	23.2_1	28.8_1	31.6_1	26.0_2	31.6_2	34.4_1	28.8_3	34.4_3	37.2_1	31.6_4	37.2_4	40.0_1	31.6_4	34.4_4	28.8_4	20.0_1
Fri																
Cycle	D/O	D/O	D/O	D/O	D/O	D/O	D/O	D/O	D/O	D/O	D/O	D/O	D/O	D/O	D/O	D/O
Sat																
Cycle	D/O	D/O	D/O	D/O	D/O	D/O	D/O	D/O	D/O	D/O	D/O	D/O	D/O	D/O	D/O	D/O
Sun																
Cycle	46.4_1	57.6_1	63.2_1	52.0_1	63.2_1	68.8_1	57.6_1	68.8_1	74.4_1	63.2_1	74.4_1	80.0_1	63.2_1	68.8_1	57.6_1	RACE

The bold subscript numerals refer to subphases; see chapter 2.

ROAD CYCLING

Race: Cycle (80 km)
Race date: 20 April
Training starts: 30 December

Maximum distance for the 100% week
Cycle: 350 km

Mileage profile

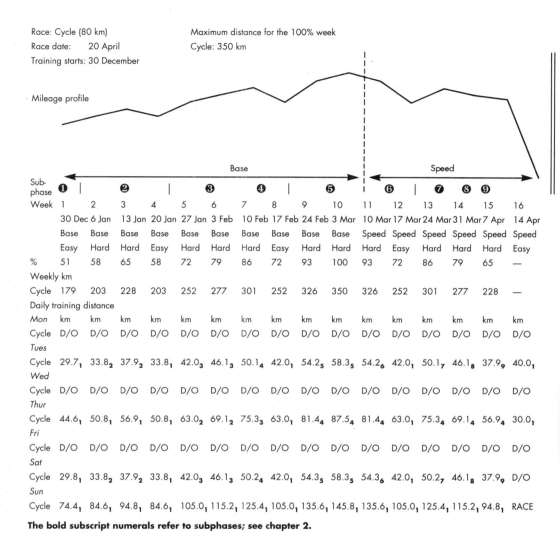

Sub-phase	❶		❷		❸	❹		❺		❻	❼	❽	❾			
	Base										Speed					
Week	1	2	3	4	5	6	7	8	9	10	11	12	13	14	15	16
	30 Dec	6 Jan	13 Jan	20 Jan	27 Jan	3 Feb	10 Feb	17 Feb	24 Feb	3 Mar	10 Mar	17 Mar	24 Mar	31 Mar	7 Apr	14 Apr
	Base	Base	Base	Base	Base	Base	Base	Base	Base	Base	Speed	Speed	Speed	Speed	Speed	Speed
	Easy	Hard	Hard	Easy	Hard	Hard	Hard	Easy	Hard	Hard	Hard	Easy	Hard	Hard	Hard	Easy
%	51	58	65	58	72	79	86	72	93	100	93	72	86	79	65	—
Weekly km																
Cycle	179	203	228	203	252	277	301	252	326	350	326	252	301	277	228	—
Daily training distance																
Mon	km	km	km	km	km	km	km	km	km	km	km	km	km	km	km	km
Cycle	D/O	D/O	D/O	D/O	D/O	D/O	D/O	D/O	D/O	D/O	D/O	D/O	D/O	D/O	D/O	D/O
Tues																
Cycle	29.7_1	33.8_2	37.9_2	33.8_1	42.0_3	46.1_3	50.1_4	42.0_1	54.2_5	58.3_5	54.2_6	42.0_1	50.1_7	46.1_8	37.9_9	40.0_1
Wed																
Cycle	D/O	D/O	D/O	D/O	D/O	D/O	D/O	D/O	D/O	D/O	D/O	D/O	D/O	D/O	D/O	D/O
Thur																
Cycle	44.6_1	50.8_1	56.9_1	50.8_1	63.0_2	69.1_2	75.3_3	63.0_1	81.4_4	87.5_4	81.4_4	63.0_1	75.3_4	69.1_4	56.9_4	30.0_1
Fri																
Cycle	D/O	D/O	D/O	D/O	D/O	D/O	D/O	D/O	D/O	D/O	D/O	D/O	D/O	D/O	D/O	D/O
Sat																
Cycle	29.8_1	33.8_2	37.9_2	33.8_1	42.0_3	46.1_3	50.2_4	42.0_1	54.3_5	58.3_5	54.3_6	42.0_1	50.2_7	46.1_8	37.9_9	D/O
Sun																
Cycle	74.4_1	84.6_1	94.8_1	84.6_1	105.0_1	115.2_1	125.4_1	105.0_1	135.6_1	145.8_1	135.6_1	105.0_1	125.4_1	115.2_1	94.8_1	RACE

The bold subscript numerals refer to subphases; see chapter 2.

Race: Cycle (80 km)
Race date: 20 April
Training starts: 30 December

Maximum distance for the 100% week
Cycle: 400 km

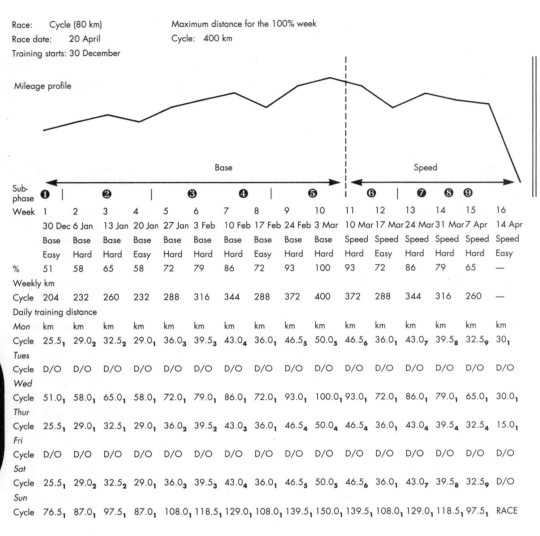

Mileage profile

Base | Speed

Sub-phase: ❶ ❷ ❸ ❹ ❺ | ❻ ❼ ❽ ❾

Week	1	2	3	4	5	6	7	8	9	10	11	12	13	14	15	16
	30 Dec	6 Jan	13 Jan	20 Jan	27 Jan	3 Feb	10 Feb	17 Feb	24 Feb	3 Mar	10 Mar	17 Mar	24 Mar	31 Mar	7 Apr	14 Apr
	Base	Base	Base	Base	Base	Base	Base	Base	Base	Base	Speed	Speed	Speed	Speed	Speed	Speed
	Easy	Hard	Hard	Easy	Hard	Hard	Hard	Easy	Hard	Hard	Hard	Easy	Hard	Hard	Hard	Easy
%	51	58	65	58	72	79	86	72	93	100	93	72	86	79	65	—
Weekly km																
Cycle	204	232	260	232	288	316	344	288	372	400	372	288	344	316	260	—
Daily training distance																
Mon	km	km	km	km	km	km	km	km	km	km	km	km	km	km	km	km
Cycle	25.5_1	29.0_2	32.5_2	29.0_1	36.0_3	39.5_3	43.0_4	36.0_1	46.5_5	50.0_5	46.5_6	36.0_1	43.0_7	39.5_8	32.5_9	30_1
Tues																
Cycle	D/O	D/O	D/O	D/O	D/O	D/O	D/O	D/O	D/O	D/O	D/O	D/O	D/O	D/O	D/O	D/O
Wed																
Cycle	51.0_1	58.0_1	65.0_1	58.0_1	72.0_1	79.0_1	86.0_1	72.0_1	93.0_1	100.0_1	93.0_1	72.0_1	86.0_1	79.0_1	65.0_1	30.0_1
Thur																
Cycle	25.5_1	29.0_1	32.5_1	29.0_1	36.0_2	39.5_2	43.0_3	36.0_1	46.5_4	50.0_4	46.5_4	36.0_1	43.0_4	39.5_4	32.5_4	15.0_1
Fri																
Cycle	D/O	D/O	D/O	D/O	D/O	D/O	D/O	D/O	D/O	D/O	D/O	D/O	D/O	D/O	D/O	D/O
Sat																
Cycle	25.5_1	29.0_2	32.5_2	29.0_1	36.0_3	39.5_3	43.0_4	36.0_1	46.5_5	50.0_5	46.5_6	36.0_1	43.0_7	39.5_8	32.5_9	D/O
Sun																
Cycle	76.5_1	87.0_1	97.5_1	87.0_1	108.0_1	118.5_1	129.0_1	108.0_1	139.5_1	150.0_1	139.5_1	108.0_1	129.0_1	118.5_1	97.5_1	RACE

Base I would occur first.

The bold subscript numerals refer to subphases; see chapter 2.

Race: Cycle (100 km)
Race date: 20 April
Training starts: 30 December

Maximum distance for the 100% week
Cycle: 500 km

Mileage profile

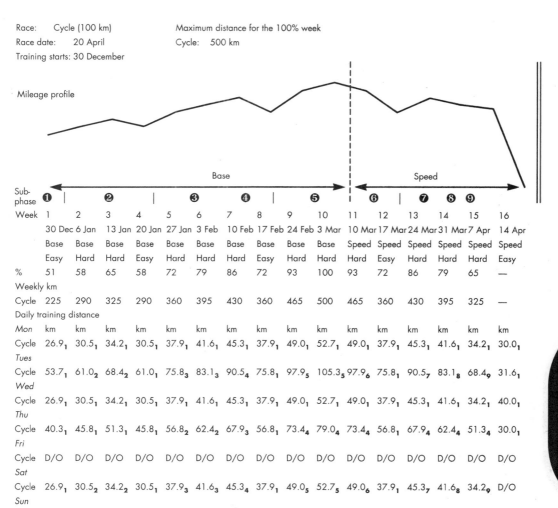

Base — Speed

Sub-phase	❶		❷		❸	❹		❺		❻		❼	❽	❾	
Week	1	2	3	4	5	6	7	8	9	10	11	12	13	14	15	16
	30 Dec	6 Jan	13 Jan	20 Jan	27 Jan	3 Feb	10 Feb	17 Feb	24 Feb	3 Mar	10 Mar	17 Mar	24 Mar	31 Mar	7 Apr	14 Apr
	Base	Base	Base	Base	Base	Base	Base	Base	Base	Base	Speed	Speed	Speed	Speed	Speed	Speed
	Easy	Hard	Hard	Easy	Hard	Hard	Hard	Easy	Hard	Hard	Hard	Easy	Hard	Hard	Hard	Easy
%	51	58	65	58	72	79	86	72	93	100	93	72	86	79	65	—
Weekly km																
Cycle	225	290	325	290	360	395	430	360	465	500	465	360	430	395	325	—

Daily training distance

Mon	km	km	km	km	km	km	km	km	km	km	km	km	km	km	km	km
Cycle	26.9_1	30.5_1	34.2_1	30.5_1	37.9_1	41.6_1	45.3_1	37.9_1	49.0_1	52.7_1	49.0_1	37.9_1	45.3_1	41.6_1	34.2_1	30.0_1
Tues																
Cycle	53.7_1	61.0_2	68.4_2	61.0_1	75.8_3	83.1_3	90.5_4	75.8_1	97.9_5	105.3_5	97.9_6	75.8_1	90.5_7	83.1_8	68.4_9	31.6_1
Wed																
Cycle	26.9_1	30.5_1	34.2_1	30.5_1	37.9_1	41.6_1	45.3_1	37.9_1	49.0_1	52.7_1	49.0_1	37.9_1	45.3_1	41.6_1	34.2_1	40.0_1
Thu																
Cycle	40.3_1	45.8_1	51.3_1	45.8_1	56.8_2	62.4_2	67.9_3	56.8_1	73.4_4	79.0_4	73.4_4	56.8_1	67.9_4	62.4_4	51.3_4	30.0_1
Fri																
Cycle	D/O	D/O	D/O	D/O	D/O	D/O	D/O	D/O	D/O	D/O	D/O	D/O	D/O	D/O	D/O	D/O
Sat																
Cycle	26.9_1	30.5_2	34.2_2	30.5_1	37.9_3	41.6_3	45.3_4	37.9_1	49.0_5	52.7_5	49.0_6	37.9_1	45.3_7	41.6_8	34.2_9	D/O
Sun																
Cycle	80.6_1	91.6_1	102.7_2	91.6_1	113.7_1	124.8_1	135.8_1	113.7_1	146.9_1	158.0_1	146.9_1	113.7_1	135.8_1	124.8_1	102.7_1	RACE

Base I would occur first.
The bold subscript numerals refer to subphases; see chapter 2.

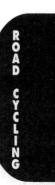

ROAD CYCLING

Race: Cycle (160 km) Maximum distance for the 100% week
Race date: 20 April Cycle: 600 km
Training starts: 30 December

Mileage profile

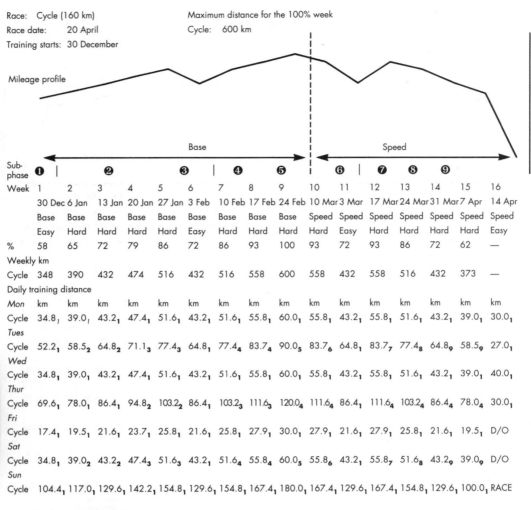

	Base									Speed						
Subphase	❶	❷		❸		❹	❺		❻	❼	❽	❾			
Week	1	2	3	4	5	6	7	8	9	10	11	12	13	14	15	16
	30 Dec	6 Jan	13 Jan	20 Jan	27 Jan	3 Feb	10 Feb	17 Feb	24 Feb	10 Mar	3 Mar	17 Mar	24 Mar	31 Mar	7 Apr	14 Apr
	Base	Base	Base	Base	Base	Base	Base	Base	Base	Speed	Speed	Speed	Speed	Speed	Speed	Speed
	Easy	Hard	Hard	Hard	Hard	Easy	Hard	Hard	Hard	Hard	Easy	Hard	Hard	Hard	Hard	Easy
%	58	65	72	79	86	72	86	93	100	93	72	93	86	72	62	—
Weekly km Cycle	348	390	432	474	516	432	516	558	600	558	432	558	516	432	373	—

Daily training distance

Day																
Mon Cycle	34.8_1	39.0_1	43.2_1	47.4_1	51.6_1	43.2_1	51.6_1	55.8_1	60.0_1	55.8_1	43.2_1	55.8_1	51.6_1	43.2_1	39.0_1	30.0_1
Tues Cycle	52.2_1	58.5_2	64.8_2	71.1_3	77.4_3	64.8_1	77.4_4	83.7_4	90.0_5	83.7_6	64.8_1	83.7_7	77.4_8	64.8_9	58.5_9	27.0_1
Wed Cycle	34.8_1	39.0_1	43.2_1	47.4_1	51.6_1	43.2_1	51.6_1	55.8_1	60.0_1	55.8_1	43.2_1	55.8_1	51.6_1	43.2_1	39.0_1	40.0_1
Thur Cycle	69.6_1	78.0_1	86.4_4	94.8_2	103.2_2	86.4_1	103.2_3	111.6_3	120.0_4	111.6_4	86.4_1	111.6_4	103.2_4	86.4_4	78.0_4	30.0_1
Fri Cycle	17.4_1	19.5_1	21.6_1	23.7_1	25.8_1	21.6_1	25.8_1	27.9_1	30.0_1	27.9_1	21.6_1	27.9_1	25.8_1	21.6_1	19.5_1	D/O
Sat Cycle	34.8_1	39.0_2	43.2_2	47.4_3	51.6_3	43.2_1	51.6_4	55.8_4	60.0_5	55.8_6	43.2_1	55.8_7	51.6_8	43.2_9	39.0_9	D/O
Sun Cycle	104.4_1	117.0_1	129.6_1	142.2_1	154.8_1	129.6_1	154.8_1	167.4_1	180.0_1	167.4_1	129.6_1	167.4_1	154.8_1	129.6_1	100.0_1	RACE

Base I would occur first.
The bold subscript numerals refer to subphases; see chapter 2.

Race: Tour (700 km)   Maximum distance for the 100% week
Race date: 20 April   Cycle: 800 km
Training starts: 30 December

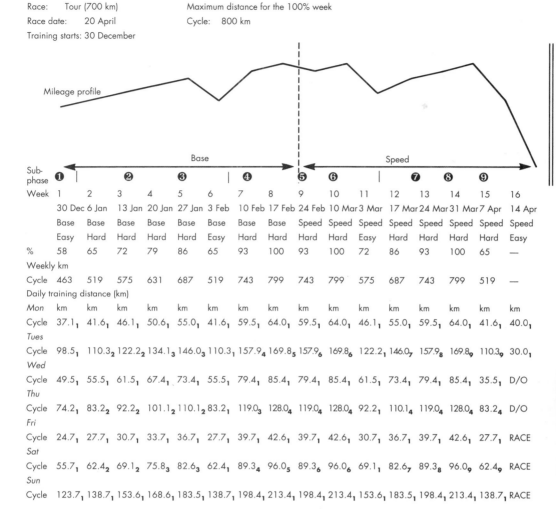

Mileage profile

Sub-phase	❶		❷		❸		❹		❺	❻		❼	❽	❾		
Week	1	2	3	4	5	6	7	8	9	10	11	12	13	14	15	16
	30 Dec	6 Jan	13 Jan	20 Jan	27 Jan	3 Feb	10 Feb	17 Feb	24 Feb	10 Mar	3 Mar	17 Mar	24 Mar	31 Mar	7 Apr	14 Apr
	Base	Base	Base	Base	Base	Base	Base	Base	Speed	Speed	Speed	Speed	Speed	Speed	Speed	Speed
	Easy	Hard	Hard	Hard	Hard	Easy	Hard	Hard	Hard	Hard	Easy	Hard	Hard	Hard	Hard	Easy
%	58	65	72	79	86	65	93	100	93	100	72	86	93	100	65	—
Weekly km Cycle	463	519	575	631	687	519	743	799	743	799	575	687	743	799	519	—

Daily training distance (km)

	Mon	Tue	Wed	Thu	Fri	Sat	Sun
	km	km	km	km	km	km	km

Mon Cycle: 37.1_1 41.6_1 46.1_1 50.6_1 55.0_1 41.6_1 59.5_1 64.0_1 59.5_1 64.0_1 46.1_1 55.0_1 59.5_1 64.0_1 41.6_1 40.0_1

Tues Cycle: 98.5_1 110.3_2 122.2_2 134.1_3 146.0_3 110.3_1 157.9_4 169.8_5 157.9_6 169.8_6 122.2_1 146.0_7 157.9_8 169.8_9 110.3_9 30.0_1

Wed Cycle: 49.5_1 55.5_1 61.5_1 67.4_1 73.4_1 55.5_1 79.4_1 85.4_1 79.4_1 85.4_1 61.5_1 73.4_1 79.4_1 85.4_1 35.5_1 D/O

Thu Cycle: 74.2_1 83.2_2 92.2_2 101.1_2 110.1_2 83.2_1 119.0_3 128.0_4 119.0_4 128.0_4 92.2_1 110.1_4 119.0_4 128.0_4 83.2_4 D/O

Fri Cycle: 24.7_1 27.7_1 30.7_1 33.7_1 36.7_1 27.7_1 39.7_1 42.6_1 39.7_1 42.6_1 30.7_1 36.7_1 39.7_1 42.6_1 27.7_1 RACE

Sat Cycle: 55.7_1 62.4_2 69.1_2 75.8_3 82.6_3 62.4_1 89.3_4 96.0_5 89.3_6 96.0_6 69.1_1 82.6_7 89.3_8 96.0_9 62.4_9 RACE

Sun Cycle: 123.7_1 138.7_1 153.6_1 168.6_1 183.5_1 138.7_1 198.4_1 213.4_1 198.4_1 213.4_1 153.6_1 183.5_1 198.4_1 213.4_1 138.7_1 RACE

Base I would occur first.

The bold subscript numerals refer to subphases; see chapter 2.

ROAD CYCLING

Race: Mountainbike

Race date: 15 Jan

Maximum distance for the 100% week

Mountainbike: 10.5 hrs (630 mins)

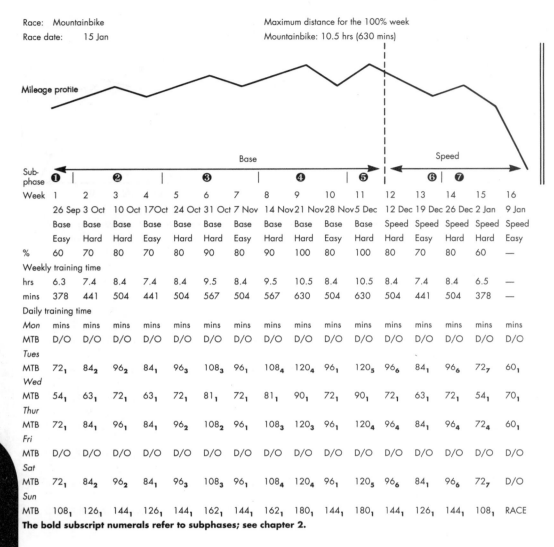

Mileage profile

Sub-phase	❶		❷		❸			❹			❺	❻	❼			
					Base							Speed				
Week	1	2	3	4	5	6	7	8	9	10	11	12	13	14	15	16
	26 Sep	3 Oct	10 Oct	17Oct	24 Oct	31 Oct	7 Nov	14 Nov	21 Nov	28 Nov	5 Dec	12 Dec	19 Dec	26 Dec	2 Jan	9 Jan
	Base	Base	Base	Base	Base	Base	Base	Base	Base	Base	Base	Speed	Speed	Speed	Speed	Speed
	Easy	Hard	Hard	Easy	Hard	Hard	Easy	Hard	Hard	Easy	Hard	Hard	Easy	Hard	Hard	Easy
%	60	70	80	70	80	90	80	90	100	80	100	80	70	80	60	—
Weekly training time																
hrs	6.3	7.4	8.4	7.4	8.4	9.5	8.4	9.5	10.5	8.4	10.5	8.4	7.4	8.4	6.5	—
mins	378	441	504	441	504	567	504	567	630	504	630	504	441	504	378	—
Daily training time																
Mon	mins	mins	mins	mins	mins	mins	mins	mins	mins	mins	mins	mins	mins	mins	mins	mins
MTB	D/O	D/O	D/O	D/O	D/O	D/O	D/O	D/O	D/O	D/O	D/O	D/O	D/O	D/O	D/O	D/O
Tues																
MTB	72_1	84_2	96_2	84_1	96_3	108_3	96_1	108_4	120_4	96_1	120_5	96_6	84_1	96_6	72_7	60_1
Wed																
MTB	54_1	63_1	72_1	63_1	72_1	81_1	72_1	81_1	90_1	72_1	90_1	72_1	63_1	72_1	54_1	70_1
Thur																
MTB	72_1	84_1	96_1	84_1	96_2	108_2	96_1	108_3	120_3	96_1	120_4	96_4	84_1	96_4	72_4	60_1
Fri																
MTB	D/O	D/O	D/O	D/O	D/O	D/O	D/O	D/O	D/O	D/O	D/O	D/O	D/O	D/O	D/O	D/O
Sat																
MTB	72_1	84_2	96_2	84_1	96_3	108_3	96_1	108_4	120_4	96_1	120_5	96_6	84_1	96_6	72_7	D/O
Sun																
MTB	108_1	126_1	144_1	126_1	144_1	162_1	144_1	162_1	180_1	144_1	180_1	144_1	126_1	144_1	108_1	RACE

The bold subscript numerals refer to subphases; see chapter 2.

MOUNTAINBIKE

Maximum distance for 100% week
Mountain bike 16 hrs (960 mins)

Mileage profile

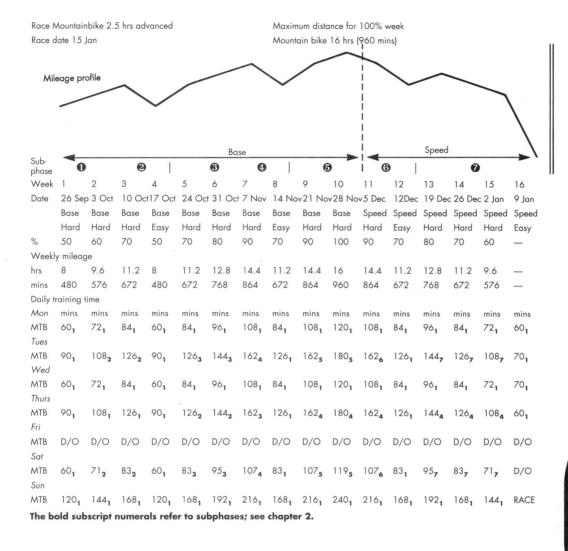

Sub-phase	❶		❷		❸		❹		❺		❻		❼			
Week	1	2	3	4	5	6	7	8	9	10	11	12	13	14	15	16
Date	26 Sep	3 Oct	10 Oct	17 Oct	24 Oct	31 Oct	7 Nov	14 Nov	21 Nov	28 Nov	5 Dec	12Dec	19 Dec	26 Dec	2 Jan	9 Jan
	Base	Base	Base	Base	Base	Base	Base	Base	Base	Base	Speed	Speed	Speed	Speed	Speed	Speed
	Hard	Hard	Hard	Easy	Hard	Hard	Hard	Easy	Hard	Hard	Hard	Easy	Hard	Hard	Hard	Easy
%	50	60	70	50	70	80	90	70	90	100	90	70	80	70	60	—
Weekly mileage																
hrs	8	9.6	11.2	8	11.2	12.8	14.4	11.2	14.4	16	14.4	11.2	12.8	11.2	9.6	—
mins	480	576	672	480	672	768	864	672	864	960	864	672	768	672	576	—
Daily training time																
Mon	mins	mins	mins	mins	mins	mins	mins	mins	mins	mins	mins	mins	mins	mins	mins	mins
MTB	60_1	72_1	84_1	60_1	84_1	96_1	108_1	84_1	108_1	120_1	108_1	84_1	96_1	84_1	72_1	60_1
Tues MTB	90_1	108_2	126_2	90_1	126_3	144_3	162_4	126_1	162_5	180_5	162_6	126_1	144_7	126_7	108_7	70_1
Wed MTB	60_1	72_1	84_1	60_1	84_1	96_1	108_1	84_1	108_1	120_1	108_1	84_1	96_1	84_1	72_1	70_1
Thurs MTB	90_1	108_1	126_1	90_1	126_2	144_2	162_3	126_1	162_4	180_4	162_4	126_1	144_4	126_4	108_4	60_1
Fri MTB	D/O	D/O	D/O	D/O	D/O	D/O	D/O	D/O	D/O	D/O	D/O	D/O	D/O	D/O	D/O	D/O
Sat MTB	60_1	71_2	83_2	60_1	83_3	95_3	107_4	83_1	107_5	119_5	107_6	83_1	95_7	83_7	71_7	D/O
Sun MTB	120_1	144_1	168_1	120_1	168_1	192_1	216_1	168_1	216_1	240_1	216_1	168_1	192_1	168_1	144_1	RACE

The bold subscript numerals refer to subphases; see chapter 2.

MOUNTAINBIKE

Spinning workouts

This chapter contains all the workouts that you can use to guide you in your 'on the road' workouts, or to use on your stationary trainer.

1. Preparation — easy training

This is easy non-specific and low-intensity training to build general endurance. You can also work on technique and check and rectify any strength imbalances.

This programme is emphasised at the start of Base training and can last 4–6 weeks (usually 2–4).

SPECIFICS: Light/easy conditioning.

EFFORT: Easy conversation pace (50–60 percent effort); easy muscular effort.

BIKE: Easy riding, mainly on the flat.
Duration: Whole workout.
During: Easy 'rolling' on the flat.
Gears: Easy/small gears — small chainring (39 or 42 x 16–21).
Cadence: 85–95 rpm for time trialling, triathlon and duathlon; 95–105 rpm for road cycling and triathlon with legal drafting.

Training heart rate = ☐

(LSD: 60–75 percent HR^{max}).
See pages 42–43 for reference table.

SPIN WORKOUT: ①   **AIM:** Easy conditioning   **TOTAL TIME:** 38 min

EXTRA INFORMATION

TRAIN TYPE	DURATION	GRAD/RES	CADENCE	EFFORT	HEART RATE	COMMENTS
Warm up	5 min	↓↓	—	Easy	LSD	Warm up
Fitness	30 s	↓↓	—	Easy	LSD	Smooth/Fluid
	30 s	—	—	Easy	LSD	Smooth/Fluid
	30 s	↑	—	Moderate	LSD	Smooth/Fluid
	30 s	↑↑	—	Moderate	LSD	Use whole pedal stroke
ILT†	1 min L	↓↓	↓↓↓	Easy	LSD	Look for strength weakness
	1 min R	↓↓	↓↓↓	Easy	LSD	Look for strength weakness
	1 min L+R	—	—	Easy	LSD	Work whole pedal stroke
	1 min L	↑	↓↓↓	Easy	LSD	
	1 min R	↑	↓↓↓	Easy	LSD	
	1 min L+R	↑↑	↓	Easy	LSD	
Positions	5 min	—	—	Easy	LSD	Aero (if tri)
	5 min	—	—	Easy	LSD	Sitting
	5 min	↑↑↑	↓↓↓	Moderate	LSD	Seated climb
	2 min	↑↑↑	↓↓↓	Moderate	LSD	Standing climb
Spin sprint	20 s*	↓↓↓	↑↑↑	Easy	LSD	Try to remain seated
	1 min	—	—	Easy	LSD	
	20 s*	↓↓↓	↑↑↑	Easy	LSD	Try to remain seated
Warm down	5 min	—	—	Easy	LSD	Relax

* Having completed the effort, pedal gently for the rest of the minute and begin the next part of the workout at the start of the next minute.

Place training heart rates from pages 42–43 in here.

† ILT = Individual leg training (see pages 51–52)

CODES	GEAR/RES	CADENCE
—	Usual/comfortable	Usual/comfortable
↑	A little harder (↑1–2 cogs)	A little higher (↑5 rpm)
↑↑	Moderately harder (↑2–3 cogs)	Moderately higher (↑10 rpm)
↑↑↑	Much harder (↑4–5 cogs)	Much higher (↑15⁺ rpm)
↓↓↓	Much easier (↓4–6 cogs)	Much lower (↓30 rpm)
↓↓	Moderately easier (↓2–4 cogs)	Moderately lower (↓20 rpm)
↓	A little easier (↓1–2 cogs)	A little lower (↓10 rpm)

SPIN WORKOUT: ①   **AIM:** Easy conditioning/ Technique   **TOTAL TIME:** 54 min
*34 min

EXTRA INFORMATION

TRAIN TYPE	DURATION	GRAD/RES	CADENCE	EFFORT	HEART RATE	COMMENTS
Warm up	5 min	—	—	Easy	LSD	
Push down	2 min	—	↓↓↓	Easy	LSD	Knees in; see pg 56
Easy	2 min	—	—	Easy	LSD	
Push down*	2 min	—	↓↓↓	Easy	LSD	Knees in; see pg 56
Easy*	2 min	—	—	Easy	LSD	
Pull up	2 min	—	↓↓↓	Easy	LSD	Use hips over top; see pg 56
Easy	2 min	—	—	Easy	LSD	
Pull up*	2 min	—	↓↓↓	Easy	LSD	Use hips over top; see pg 56
Easy*	2 min	—	—	Easy	LSD	
Big gear	1 min	↑↑↑	↓↓↓	Easy	LSD	see pg 57
Little gear	1 min	↓↓↓	↑↑↑	Easy	LSD	see pg 57
Easy	2 min	—	—	Easy	LSD	
Big gear*	1 min	↑↑↑	↓↓↓	Easy	LSD	see pg 57
Little gear*	1 min	~ ↓↓↓	↑↑↑	Easy	LSD	see pg 57
Easy*	2 min	—	—	Easy	LSD	
Scrape mud	2 min	—	↓↓↓	Easy	LSD	Pull back use calf; see pg 56
Easy*	2 min	—	—	Easy	LSD	
Scrape mud*	2 min	—	↓↓↓	Easy	LSD	Pull back use calf; see pg 56
Easy*	2 min	—	—	Easy	LSD	
U/K*	2 min	—	↓↓↓	Easy	LSD	Use hips to lift; see pg 56
Easy*	2 min	—	—	Easy	LSD	
U/K	2 min	—	↓↓↓	Easy	LSD	Use hips to lift; see pg 56
Easy	2 min	—	—	Easy	LSD	
Wind handle	2 min	—	—	Easy	LSD	Combination; see pg 56
Big gear	1 min	↑↑↑	↓↓↓	Easy	LSD	See pg 57
Little gear	1 min	↓↓↓	↑↑↑	Easy	LSD	See pg 57
Warm down	5 min	—	—	Easy	LSD	

* Remove these parts of your programme for a shorter/easier workout.

Place training heart rates from pages 42–43 in here.

U/K = Up and kick door

CODES	GEAR/RES	CADENCE
—	Usual/comfortable	Usual/comfortable
↑	A little harder (↑1–2 cogs)	A little higher (↑5 rpm)
↑↑	Moderately harder (↑2–3 cogs)	Moderately higher (↑10 rpm)
↑↑↑	Much harder (↑4–5 cogs)	Much higher (↑15⁺ rpm)
↓↓↓	Much easier (↓4–6 cogs)	Much lower (↓30 rpm)
↓↓	Moderately easier (↓2–4 cogs)	Moderately lower (↓20 rpm)
↓	A little easier (↓1–2 cogs)	A little lower (↓10 rpm)

SPIN WORKOUT: Sub ①   **AIM:** Easy conditioning/ Technique   **TOTAL TIME:** 85 min *39 min

EXTRA INFORMATION

TRAIN TYPE	DURATION	GRAD/RES	CADENCE	EFFORT	HEART RATE	COMMENTS
Warm up	5 min	—	—	Easy	LSD	
Endurance	10 min	—	—	Easy	LSD	
Overspeed	10 s†					See pg 134
Push down	3 min	↑	↓	Easy	LSD	Knees in; see pg 56
Overspeed*	10 s†	↓↓↓	↑↑↑	Easy	N/A	
Endurance*	10 min	—	—	Easy	LSD	
Overspeed*	10 s†	↓↓↓	↑↑↑	Easy	N/A	
Pull up	3 min	↑	↓	Easy	LSD	Use hips over to; see pg 56
Overspeed	10 s†	↓↓↓	↑↑↑	Easy	N/A	
Endurance*	10 min	—	—	Easy	LSD	
Overspeed*	10 s†	↓↓↓	↑↑↑	Easy	N/A	
Scrape mud	3 min	↑	↓	Easy	LSD	Pull back use calf; see pg 56
Overspeed*	10 s†	↓↓↓	↑↑↑	Easy	N/A	
Endurance*	10 min	—	—	Easy	LSD	
Overspeed*	10 s†	↓↓↓	↑↑↑	Easy	N/A	
U/K	3 min	↑	↓	Easy	LSD	Ue hips to lift; see pg 56
Overspeed	10 s†	↓↓↓	↑↑↑	Easy	N/A	
Endurance*	10 min	—	—	Easy	LSD	
Overspeed*	10 s†	↓↓↓	↑↑↑	Easy	N/A	
Wind handle	3 min	↑	↓	Easy	LSD	Combination; see pg 56
Overspeed	10 s†	↓↓↓	↑↑↑	Easy	N/A	
Warm down	5 min	—	—	Easy	LSD	Relax

U/K = Up and kick door

Place training heart rates from page 42–43 in here.

* Remove these parts of your programme for a shorter/easier workout.

† Having completed the effort, pedal gently for the rest of the minute and begin the next part of the workout at the start of the next minute.

CODES	GEAR/RES	CADENCE
—	Usual/comfortable	Usual/comfortable
↑	A little harder (↑1–2 cogs)	A little higher (↑5 rpm)
↑↑	Moderately harder (↑2–3 cogs)	Moderately higher (↑10 rpm)
↑↑↑	Much harder (↑4–5 cogs)	Much higher (↑15+ rpm)
↓↓↓	Much easier (↓4–6 cogs)	Much lower (↓30 rpm)
↓↓	Moderately easier (↓2–4 cogs)	Moderately lower (↓20 rpm)
↓	A little easier (↓1–2 cogs)	A little lower (↓10 rpm)

SPIN WORKOUT: Sub ① **AIM:** Easy conditioning/Technique **TOTAL TIME:** 40–53 min

EXTRA INFORMATION

TRAIN TYPE	SET	REP	DURATION	REST*	GEAR	CADENCE	GRAD/RES	HEART RATE	COMMENTS
Warm up	3-6x	1x	20 s	—	42 x 18-21	75-85	0% or 1	LSD	Easy
		1x	20 s	—	42 x 18-21	85-95	0% or 1	LSD	Easy
		1x	10 s	—	42 x 18-21	95-105	0% or 1	LSD	Easy
		1x	10 s	—	42 x 18-21	105-125	0% or 1	LSD	Easy
Fitness	2-4x	1x	30 s	—	42 x 18-21	85-95	0% or 1	LSD	Smooth fluid pedalling
		1x	30 s	—	42 x 16-18	85-95	0% or 1	LSD	Smooth fluid pedalling
		1x	30 s	—	42 x 14-16	85-95	0% or 1	LSD	Smooth fluid pedalling
		1x	30 s	—	42 x 12-14	85-95	0% or 1	LSD	Use whole pedal stroke
ILT	2-4x	1x	1 min L	—	42 x 18-21	60-80	0% or 1	LSD	Look for weakness
		1x	1 min R	—	42 x 18-21	60-80	0% or 1	LSD	Look for weakness
		1x	1 min L+R	—	42 x 18-21	60-80	0% or 1	LSD	Work whole pedal stroke
Positions	1x	1x	5 min	—	42 x 14-18	85-95	0% or 1	LSD	Aero position
		1x	5 min	—	42 x 14-18	85-95	0% or 1	LSD	Seated
		1x	5 min	—	52 x 12	60-70	3-5% or 3-4	N/A	Seated climb
		1x	2 min	—	52 x 12	60-70	5-7% or 4-6	N/A	Standing climb
Spin sprint	—	3x	20 s	1 min	42 x 18	120+	0% or 1	N/A	Try to remain seated
Warm down	—	1x	5 min	—	42 x 18-21	85-95	0% or 1	LSD	Easy

Place training heart rates from pages 42–43 in here.

* Rest means easy active recovery pedalling (42 x 18–21).

SPIN WORKOUT: Sub ①   **AIM:** Endurance/Technique (1)   **TOTAL TIME:** 42–60 min

EXTRA INFORMATION

GEAR	CADENCE	GRAD/RES	HEART RATE	COMMENTS
42 x 18	85–95	0% or 1	LSD	Easy
42 x 16	85–95	0% or 1	LSD	Easy
42 x 14	85–95	0% or 1	LSD	Easy
42 x 18	85–95	0% or 1	LSD	Easy
42 x 18	95–105	0% or 1	LSD	Relax hips
42 x 18	105–120	0% or 1	LSD	Relax hips
42 x 16	85–95	0% or 1	LSD	Knees in; see pg 56
42 x 16	85–95	0% or 1	LSD	Use hips over top; see pg 56
42 x 16	85–95	0% or 1	LSD	Pull back use calf; see pg 56
42 x 16	85–95	0% or 1	LSD	Use hips to lift; see pg 56
42 x 16	85–95	0% or 1	LSD	Combination; see pg 56
42 x 18	95+	0% or 1	LSD	Relax/smooth/fluid; see pg 57
52 x 12	40–60	3–5% or 3–4	N/A	Use whole pedal stroke
42 x 18	85–95	0% or 1	LSD	Easy

Place training heart rates from pages 42–43 in here.

TRAIN TYPE	SET	REP	DURATION	REST*
Warm up	1x	1x	1 min	—
		1x	1 min	—
		1x	1 min	—
		1x	1 min	—
Spin	—	1x	1 min	2 min
Spin	—	1x	1 min	2 min
Push down	—	1x	2 min	2 min
Pull up	—	1-2x	1 min	2 min
Scrape mud	—	1-3x	1 min	2 min
U/K	—	1-3x	1 min	2 min
Wind handle	—	1 x	2-5 min	—
BG/LG	4x	1x	1 min	—
		1x	1 min	1 min
Warm down	—	1x	5 min	—

U/K Up and kick door

*Rest means easy active recovery pedalling (42 x 18–21).

SPIN WORKOUT: Sub ① **AIM:** Easy conditioning/Technique   **TOTAL TIME:** 85 min

EXTRA INFORMATION

TRAIN TYPE	SET	REP	DURATION	REST	GEAR	CADENCE	GRAD/RES	HEART RATE	COMMENTS
Warm up	—	1x	5 min	—	42 x 16–21	85–95	0%	LSD	Easy
Endurance	—	1x	10 min	—	42 x 15–18	85–95	0%	LSD	Easy
Push down	—	1x	5 min	—	42 x 12–16	60–70	0%	N/A	Knees in; see pg 56
Endurance	—	1x	10 min	—	42 x 15–18	85–95	0%	LSD	Easy
Pull up	—	1x	5 min	—	42 x 12–16	60–70	0%	N/A	Use hips over top; see pg 56
Endurance	—	1x	10 min	—	42 x 15–18	85–95	0%	LSD	Easy
Scrape mud	—	1x	5 min	—	42 x 12–16	60–70	0%	N/A	Pull back use calf; see pg 56
Endurance	—	1x	10 min	—	42 x 15–18	85–95	0%	LSD	Easy
U/K	—	1x	5 min	—	42 x 12–16	60–70	0%	N/A	Use hips to lift; see pg 56
Endurance	—	1x	10 min	—	42 x 15–18	85–95	0%	LSD	Easy
Wind handle	—	1x	5 min	—	42 x 12–16	60–70	3–5%	N/A	Combination; see pg 57
Warm down	—	1x	5 min	—	42 x 16–21	85–95	0%	LSD	Easy

Place training heart rates from page 42–43 in here.

U/K Up and kick door

2. Load training — hill training

Load training involves incorporating hills into your training programme. This brings in strength endurance training, which is the start of training your body to push a bigger gear when racing. Load is emphasised in early Base, and would occur progressively from once to twice a week. This phase could last from 2–8 weeks (generally 4).

SPECIFICS: Strength endurance training. Steady climbs on the hills at low pedal cadence.

EFFORT: *During:* Medium effort (65–75 percent); medium muscular effort.

Between: Easy conversation pace (50–60 percent effort); easy muscular effort.

BIKE: Hills (easy gears) — small to big hills.
Duration: Whole workout.
During: On the hills.
Gears: Easy/small gears (39 or 42 x 18–21).
Cadence: 40–60 rpm.
Between: On the flat.
Gears: Easy/small gears — small chainring (39 or 42 x 16–21).
Cadence: 85–95 rpm for time trialling, triathlon and duathlon; 95–105 rpm for road cycling and triathlon with legal drafting.

Training heart rate = During: N/A   Between:
(LSD: 60–75 percent HR^{max}).
See pages 42–43 for reference table.

Simulating hills on a stationary trainer

There are two ways to incorporate hills:

1. Alternate small with bigger gears on your trainer (e.g. 52 or 53 x 16–21 to simulate hills, and 39–42 x 16–21 to rest in between to simulate the flat);

2. If you have a stationary trainer with an adjustable resistance or gradient, adjust the resistance to be harder (higher resistance or 3–5 percent gradient) to simulate hills and lower the resistance (0 percent gradient) to simulate the flat.

PROGRAMME 2A   INTERMEDIATE SPORT

2

SPIN WORKOUT: Sub ② (1,2)   **AIM:** Strength endurance   **TOTAL TIME:** 65 min *30 min

EXTRA INFORMATION

TRAIN TYPE	DURATION	GRAD/RES	CADENCE	EFFORT	HEART RATE	COMMENTS
Warm up	5 min	—	—	Easy	LSD	
Easy	2 min	—	—	Easy	LSD	
Hills	2 min	↑↑	↓↓	Grunt	N/A	Seated
Easy*	2 min	—	—	Easy	LSD	
Hills*	3 min	↑↑	↓↓	Grunt	N/A	Seated
Easy	2 min	—	—	Easy	LSD	
Hills	2 min	↑	↓	Grunt	N/A	Seated
Hills	2 min	↑↑	↓↓	Grunt	N/A	Standing
Easy	2 min	—	—	Easy	LSD	
Hills	2 min	↑↑	↓↓	Grunt	N/A	Seated
Hills BG*	3 min	↑↑↑	↓↓↓	Grunt	N/A	BG = Big Gear, see pg 96
Hills*	2 min	↑↑	↓↓	Grunt	N/A	Seated
Hills BG*	3 min	↑↑↑	↓↓↓	Grunt	N/A	Standing
Easy*	2 min	—	—	Easy	LSD	
Hills*	1 min	↑	↓	Grunt	N/A	Seated
Hills*	1 min	↑↑	↓↓	Grunt	N/A	
Hills BG*	1 min	↑↑↑	↓↓↓	Grunt	N/A	
Easy*	3 min	—	—	Easy	LSD	
Hills*	2 min	↑	↓	Grunt	N/A	Seated
Easy*	2 min	—	—	Easy	LSD	
Hills*	4 min	↑↑	↓↓	Grunt	N/A	Standing
Easy	2 min	—	—	Easy	LSD	
Hills	2 min	↑	↓	Grunt	N/A	Seated
Hills	2 min	↑↑	↓↓	Grunt	N/A	
Hills BG*	2 min	↑↑↑	↓↓↓	Grunt	N/A	
Hills*	2 min	↑↑	↓↓	Grunt	N/A	Standing
Hills BG*	2 min	↑↑↑	↓↓↓	Grunt	N/A	
Warm down	5 min	—	—	Easy	LSD	

Place training heart rates from pages 42–43 in here.

CODES	GEAR/RES	CADENCE
—	Usual/comfortable	Usual/comfortable
↑	A little harder (↑1–2 cogs)	A little higher (↑5 rpm)
↑↑	Moderately harder (↑2–3 cogs)	Moderately higher (↑10 rpm)
↑↑↑	Much harder (↑4–5 cogs)	Much higher (↑15+ rpm)
↓↓↓	Much easier (↓4–6 cogs)	Much lower (↓30 rpm)
↓↓	Moderately easier (↓2–4 cogs)	Moderately lower (↓20 rpm)
↓	A little easier (↓1–2 cogs)	A little lower (↓10 rpm)

* Remove these parts of your programme for a shorter/easier workout.

SPIN WORKOUT: Sub ② (1,2,3)   **AIM:** Strength endurance   **TOTAL TIME:** 73 min *43 min

EXTRA INFORMATION

TRAIN TYPE	DURATION	GRAD/RES	CADENCE	EFFORT	HEART RATE	COMMENTS
Warm up	5 min	↓↓	—	Easy	LSD	
Easy	5 min	—	—	Easy	LSD	
Hills	1 min	↑	↓	Grunt	N/A	Seated
Easy	1 min	—	—	Easy	LSD	
Hills	2 min	↑	↓	Grunt	N/A	Standing
Easy	1 min	↓↓	↑↑	Easy	N/A	
Hills*	4 min	↑↑	↓↓	Grunt	N/A	Seated
Easy*	2 min	—	—	Easy	LSD	
Hills	2 min	↑	↓	Grunt	N/A	Standing
Easy*	4 min	—	—	Easy	LSD	
Hills*	6 min	↑	↓	Grunt	N/A	Seated
Easy	1 min	—	—	Easy	LSD	
Hills	2 min	↑↑	↓↓	Grunt	N/A	Standing
Easy*	2 min	↓↓	↑↑	Easy	N/A	
Hills*	4 min	↑↑	↓↓	Grunt	N/A	Seated
Easy	3 min	—	—	Easy	LSD	
Hills	2 min	↑↑	↓↓	Grunt	N/A	Standing
Easy*	2 min	—	—	Easy	LSD	
Hills*	4 min	↑	↓	Grunt	N/A	Seated
Easy*	1 min	—	—	Easy	LSD	
Hills BG*	1 min	↑↑↑	↓↓↓	Grunt	N/A	BG = Big Gear, see pg 96
Easy	2 min	—	—	Easy	LSD	
Hills	3 min	↑↑	↓↓	Grunt	N/A	Standing
Easy	3 min	—	—	Easy	LSD	
Hills	2 min	↑	↓	Grunt	N/A	Seated
Easy	2 min	—	—	Easy	LSD	
Hills	1 min	↑↑	↓↓	Grunt	N/A	Seated
Warm down	5 min	—	—	Easy	LSD	

CODES	GEAR/RES	CADENCE
—	Usual/comfortable	Usual/comfortable
↑	A little harder (↑1–2 cogs)	A little higher (↑5 rpm)
↑↑	Moderately harder (↑2–3 cogs)	Moderately higher (↑10 rpm)
↑↑↑	Much harder (↑4–5 cogs)	Much higher (↑15+ rpm)
↓↓↓	Much easier (↓4–6 cogs)	Much lower (↓30 rpm)
↓↓	Moderately easier (↓2–4 cogs)	Moderately lower (↓20 rpm)
↓	A little easier (↓1–2 cogs)	A little lower (↓10 rpm)

Place training heart rates from pages 42–43 in here.

* Remove these parts of your programme for a shorter/easier workout.

PROGRAMME 2C

INTERMEDIATE SPORT

SPIN WORKOUT: Sub ②
(1,2,5,6,9)

AIM: Strength endurance

TOTAL TIME: 65 min
*36 min

EXTRA INFORMATION

TRAIN TYPE	DURATION	GRAD/RES	CADENCE	EFFORT	HEART RATE	COMMENTS
Warm up	5 min	—	—	Easy	LSD	
Overspeed*	10 s†	↓↓↓	↑↑↑	Easy	N/A	See pg 134
Easy*	2 min	—	—	Easy	LSD	
Overspeed*	10 s†	↓↓↓	↑↑↑	Easy	N/A	
Easy*	2 min	—	—	Easy	LSD	
AT*	3 min	—	—	Hard	AT	See pg 117
Easy*	3 min	—	—	Easy	LSD	
Tempo*	3 min	—	—	Tempo	UT	See pg 110
Easy*	3 min	—	—	Easy	LSD	
Overspeed*	10 s†	↓↓↓	↑↑↑	Easy	N/A	
Easy*	10 min	—	—	Easy	LSD	
Hills	3 min	↑↑	↓↓	Grunt	N/A	
Overspeed	10 s†	↓↓↓	↑↑↑	Easy	N/A	
Easy	10 min	—	—	Easy	LSD	
Hills	6 min	↑↑	↓↓	Grunt	N/A	
Overspeed	10 s†	↓↓↓	↑↑↑	Easy	N/A	
Warm down	10 min	—	—	Easy	LSD	

> Place training heart rates from pages 42–43 in here.

* Remove these parts of your programme for a shorter/easier workout.

† Having completed the effort, pedal gently for the rest of the minute and begin the next part of the workout at the start of the next minute.

CODES	GEAR/RES	CADENCE
—	Usual/comfortable	Usual/comfortable
↑	A little harder (↑1–2 cogs)	A little higher (↑5 rpm)
↑↑	Moderately harder (↑2–3 cogs)	Moderately higher (↑10 rpm)
↑↑↑	Much harder (↑4–5 cogs)	Much higher (↑15+ rpm)
↓↓↓	Much easier (↓4–6 cogs)	Much lower (↓30 rpm)
↓↓	Moderately easier (↓2–4 cogs)	Moderately lower (↓20 rpm)
↓	A little easier (↓1–2 cogs)	A little lower (↓10 rpm)

SPIN WORKOUT: Sub ②   **AIM:** Strength endurance   **TOTAL TIME:** 26–66 min

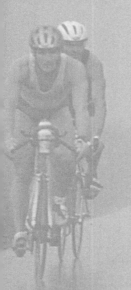

TRAIN TYPE	SET	REP	DURATION	REST*
Warm up	2x	1x	1 min	—
		1x	1 min	—
		1x	1 min	—
		1x	1 min	—
Hills	—	6–10x	1–3 min	2 min
Warm down	2x	1x	1 min	—
		1x	1 min	—
		1x	30s	—
		1x	30s	—

EXTRA INFORMATION

	GEAR	CADENCE	GRAD/RES	HEART RATE	COMMENTS
	42 x 18–21	85–95	0% or 1	LSD	Easy
	42 x 16–18	85–95	0% or 1	LSD	Easy
	42 x 14–16	85–95	0% or 1	LSD	Easy
	42 x 18–21	85–95	0% or 1	LSD	Easy
	42 x 14–16	40–60	3–5% or 3–4	N/A	Grunt; alternate seated and standing
	42 x 14–16	85–95	0% or 1	LSD	Easy
	42 x 14–16	95–105	0% or 1	LSD	Easy
	42 x 14–16	85–95	0% or 1	LSD	Easy
	42 x 14–16	105+	0% or 1	LSD	Easy

Place training heart rates from pages 42–43 in here.

* Rest means easy active recovery pedalling (42 x 18–21).

SPIN WORKOUT: Sub ② (1,2,4) **AIM:** Strength endurance **TOTAL TIME:** 55–99 min

TRAIN TYPE	SET	REP	DURATION	REST*	GEAR	CADENCE	GRAD/RES	HEART RATE	COMMENTS
Warm up	—	1x	5–10 min	—	42 x 18–21	85–95	0% or 1	LSD	Easy
Endurance	—	1x	5 min	—	42 x 14–16	85–95	0% or 1	LSD	Easy
Hills	—	1x	5 min	—	42 x 14–16	40–60	3% or 3	N/A	Grunt; long climb seated
Endurance	—	1x	5 min	—	42 x 14–16	85–95	0% or 1	LSD	Easy
Hills	—	1x	3–10 min	—	42 x 14–16	40–60	3% or 3	N/A	Long climb ½ seated
Endurance	—	1x	5 min	—	42 x 14–16	85–95	0% or 1	LSD	Easy
Flat BG	1-2x	1x	10 min	—	53 x 12–16	60–65	0% or 1	N/A	Grunt; BG = Big Gear; see pg 103
	—	1x	5 min	—	53 x 12–16	70–75	0% or 1	N/A	Grunt
	—	1x	2 min	5–10 min	53 x 12–16	80–85	0% or 1	N/A	Grunt
Warm down	—	1x	5 min	—	42 x 18–21	85–95	0% or 1	LSD	Easy

EXTRA INFORMATION

Place training heart rates from page 42–43 in here.

* **Rest means easy active recovery pedalling (42 x 18-21).**

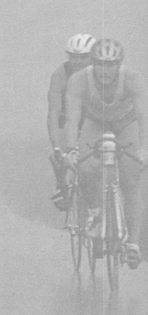

SPIN WORKOUT: Sub ② (1,2,3)   **AIM:** Strength endurance   **TOTAL TIME:** 30–90 min

TRAIN TYPE	SET	REP	DURATION	REST*	GEAR	CADENCE	GRAD/RES	HEART RATE	COMMENTS
Warm up	1x	1x	1 min	—	42 x 18	85-95	0% or 1	LSD	Aim to be only slightly 'puffing'
		1x	1 min	—	42 x 16	85-95	0% or 1	LSD	
		1x	1 min	—	42 x 14	85-95	0% or 1	LSD	
		1x	1 min	—	42 x 18	85-95	0% or 1	LSD	
Hills	—	4-10x	1 min	2 min	42 x 16-12	60-70	3% or 3	N/A	Seated hills alternating with standing hills for strength end.
Hills BG	—	1-4x	1 min	3 min	52 x 20-18	40-65	5-7% or 4-6	N/A	Loaded strength endurance BG = Big Gear, pg 96
Warm down	—	1x	10-40 min	—	42 x 114-16	85-95	0% or 1	LSD	Easy endurance

EXTRA INFORMATION

Place training heart rates from page 42–43 in here.

* Rest means easy active recovery pedalling (42 x 18-21).

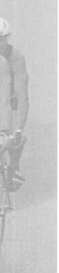

2

3. High load – hills, big-gear training

High-load training uses higher loads than can be generated by climbing hills. Further resistance is added by using bigger gears. This is a further extension of strength endurance training. It is very important that you have a coach to guide you through this.

This training is emphasised in the middle of Base. It would occur from not at all to once or twice a week over a 2–8-week period (generally 4 weeks).

SPECIFICS: High strength endurance. Steady climbs on the hills in big gears at low pedal cadence.

EFFORT: *During:* Medium effort (75–85 percent); high muscular effort.

      Between: Easy conversation pace (50–60 percent effort); easy muscular effort.

BIKE: Hills (big gears): small to big hills.

      Duration: Usually 200–700-metre reps.

            During: On the hills.

            Gears: Medium/big gears (1–5 cogs higher than you would usually use on a particular hill);

            39 or 42 x 12–16 for most people;

            52 or 53 x 12–16 for top athletes.

            Cadence: 40–60 rpm.

      Between: On the flat.

            Gears: Easy/small gears — small chainring (39 or 42 x 16–21).

            Cadence: 85–95 rpm for time trialling, triathlon and duathlon; 95–105 rpm for road cycling and triathlon with legal drafting.

Training heart rate = During: N/A   Between:

                          LSD: 60–75 percent HR^{max}).

                      See pages 42–43 for reference table.

Simulating hills on a stationary trainer

There are two ways to put hills in:

1. Alternate small with bigger gears on your trainer (e.g. 52 or 53 x 16–21 to simulate hills, and 39–42 x 16–21 to rest in between to simulate the flat);

2. If you have a stationary trainer with an adjustable resistance or gradient, adjust the resistance to be harder (higher resistance or 7–10 percent gradient) to simulate hills and lower the resistance (0 percent gradient) to simulate the flat. In this situation you just apply more resistance.

SPIN WORKOUT: Sub ③
(1,2,3)

AIM: High strength endurance

TOTAL TIME: 62 min
*37 min

EXTRA INFORMATION

TRAIN TYPE	DURATION	GRAD/RES	CADENCE	EFFORT	HEART RATE	COMMENTS
Warm up	5 min	—	—	Easy	LSD	
Hills	4 min	↑	↓	Grunt	N/A	
Easy	5 min	—	—	Easy	LSD	
Hills*	4 min	↑↑	↓↓	Grunt	N/A	
Easy*	5 min	—	—	Easy	LSD	
Hills BG	2 min	↑↑↑	↓↓↓	Grunt	N/A	BG = Big Gear
Easy	5 min	—	—	Easy	LSD	
Hills BG*	2 min	↑↑↑	↓↓↓	Grunt	N/A	
Easy*	5 min	—	—	Easy	LSD	
Hills BG	4 min	↑↑↑	↓↓↓	Grunt	N/A	
Easy	5 min	—	—	Easy	LSD	
Hills BG*	4 min	↑↑↑	↓↓↓	Grunt	N/A	
Easy*	5 min	—	—	Easy	LSD	
Hills BG	2 min	↑↑↑	↓↓↓	Grunt	N/A	
Warm down	5 min	—	—	Easy	LSD	

* Remove these parts of your programme for a shorter/easier workout.

Place training heart rates from page 42–43 in here.

CODES	GEAR/RES	CADENCE
—	Usual/comfortable	Usual/comfortable
↑	A little harder (↑1–2 cogs)	A little higher (↑5 rpm)
↑↑	Moderately harder (↑2–3 cogs)	Moderately higher (↑10 rpm)
↑↑↑	Much harder (↑4–5 cogs)	Much higher (↑15⁺ rpm)
↓↓↓	Much easier (↓4–6 cogs)	Much lower (↓30 rpm)
↓↓	Moderately easier (↓2–4 cogs)	Moderately lower (↓20 rpm)
↓	A little easier (↓1–2 cogs)	A little lower (↓10 rpm)

SPIN WORKOUT: Sub ③
(1,2,3)

AIM: High strength endurance

TOTAL TIME: 67 min
*43 min

EXTRA INFORMATION

TRAIN TYPE	DURATION	GRAD/RES	CADENCE	EFFORT	HEART RATE	COMMENTS
Warm up	5 min	—	—	Easy	LSD	
Hills*	2 min	↑	↓	Grunt	N/A	
Easy*	2 min	—	—	Easy	LSD	
Hills	3 min	↑	↓	Grunt	N/A	
Easy	2 min	—	—	Easy	LSD	
Hills	4 min	↑↑	↓↓	Grunt	N/A	
Easy	2 min	—	—	Easy	LSD	
Hills BG	2 min	↑↑↑	↓↓↓	Grunt	N/A	BG = Big Gear
Easy	4 min	—	—	Easy	LSD	
Hills BG*	2 min	↑↑↑	↓↓↓	Grunt	N/A	
Easy*	4 min	—	—	Easy	LSD	
Hills BG	4 min	↑↑↑	↓↓↓	Grunt	N/A	
Easy	4 min	—	—	Easy	LSD	
Hills	2 min	↑	↓	Grunt	N/A	
Hills BG	2 min	↑↑↑	↓↓↓	Grunt	N/A	
Easy	4 min	—	—	Easy	LSD	
Hills*	2 min	↑↑	↓↓	Grunt	N/A	
Hills BG*	2 min	↑↑↑	↓↓↓	Grunt	N/A	
Easy*	4 min	—	—	Easy	LSD	
Hills*	2 min	↑↑	↓↓	Grunt	N/A	
Hills BG*	2 min	↑↑↑	↓↓↓	Grunt	N/A	
Hills*	2 min	↑↑	↓↓	Grunt	N/A	
Warm down	5 min	—	—	Easy	LSD	

*** Remove these parts of your programme
for a shorter/easier workout.**

Place training heart rates
from page 42–43 in here.

CODES	GEAR/RES	CADENCE
—	Usual/comfortable	Usual/comfortable
↑	A little harder (↑1–2 cogs)	A little higher (↑5 rpm)
↑↑	Moderately harder (↑2–3 cogs)	Moderately higher (↑10 rpm)
↑↑↑	Much harder (↑4–5 cogs)	Much higher (↑15+ rpm)
↓↓↓	Much easier (↓4–6 cogs)	Much lower (↓30 rpm)
↓↓	Moderately easier (↓2–4 cogs)	Moderately lower (↓20 rpm)
↓	A little easier (↓1–2 cogs)	A little lower (↓10 rpm)

SPIN WORKOUT: Sub ③ **AIM:** High strength endurance **TOTAL TIME:** 70 min
(1,2,3,5,6,7,9)   /Speed endurance   *42 min

3

EXTRA INFORMATION

TRAIN TYPE	DURATION	GRAD/RES	CADENCE	EFFORT	HEART RATE	COMMENTS
Warm up	5 min	—	—	Easy	LSD	
Flat sprint*	30 s†	—	—	V Hard	N/A	#
Easy*	2 min	—	—	Easy	LSD	# **Non-drafting, time trials,**
Crest sprint*	30 s†	↑	↓	V Hard	N/A	# **triathlon, duathlon,**
Easy*	2 min	—	—	Easy	LSD	# **mountainbiking and**
Uphill sprint*	30 s†	↑↑	↓↓	V Hard	N/A	# **multisport to exclude.**
Easy*	2 min	—	—	Easy	LSD	See pg 123 for explanation of sprints
AT*	2 min	—	—	Hard	AT	See pg 117
Easy*	2 min	—	—	Easy	LSD	
Tempo*	4 min	—	—	Tempo	UT	See pg 110
Easy	2 min	—	—	Easy	LSD	
Hills	2 min	↑	↓	Grunt	N/A	
Easy	2 min	—	—	Easy	LSD	
Hills	2 min	↑↑	↓↓	Grunt	N/A	
Hills BG	2 min	↑↑↑	↓↓↓	Grunt	N/A	BG = Big Gear
Easy	4 min	—	—	Easy	LSD	
Hills	2 min	↑↑	↓↓	Grunt	N/A	
Hills BG	2 min	↑↑↑	↓↓↓	Grunt	N/A	
Hills*	2 min	↑↑	↓↓	Grunt	N/A	
Easy	4 min	—	—	Easy	LSD	
Hills	2 min	↑	↓	Grunt	N/A	
Hills BG	2 min	↑↑↑	↓↓↓	Grunt	N/A	
Overspeed	10 s†	↓↓↓	↑↑↑	Grunt	N/A	See pg 134
Easy*	4 min	—	—	Easy	LSD	
Hill*	2 min	↑↑	↓↓	Grunt	N/A	
Hills BG*	2 min	↑↑↑	↓↓↓	Grunt	N/A	
Overspeed*	10 s†	↓↓↓	↑↑↑	Grunt	N/A	
Warm down	10 min	—	—	Easy	LSD	

* Remove these parts of your programme for a shorter/easier workout.

† Having completed the effort, pedal gently for the rest of the minute and begin the next part of the workout at the start of the next minute.

Place training heart rates from page 42–43 in here.

CODES	GEAR/RES	CADENCE
—	Usual/comfortable	Usual/comfortable
↑	A little harder (↑1–2 cogs)	A little higher (↑5 rpm)
↑↑	Moderately harder (↑2–3 cogs)	Moderately higher (↑10 rpm)
↑↑↑	Much harder (↑4–5 cogs)	Much higher (↑15⁺ rpm)
↓↓↓	Much easier (↓4–6 cogs)	Much lower (↓30 rpm)
↓↓	Moderately easier (↓2–4 cogs)	Moderately lower (↓20 rpm)
↓	A little easier (↓1–2 cogs)	A little lower (↓10 rpm)

SPIN WORKOUT: Sub ③ (1,2,3)   **AIM:** High strength endurance   **TOTAL TIME:** 24–64 min

TRAIN TYPE	SET	REP	DURATION	REST**	GEAR	CADENCE	GRAD/RES	HEART RATE	COMMENTS
Warm up	—	1x	5 min	—	42 x 16–21	85–95	0% or 1	LSD	Easy
Hills	—	1–2x	1–2 min	2 min	42 x 14–16	40–60	3% or 3	N/A	Seated
Hills BG	—	1–2x	1–2 min	3 min	42 x 12–14	40–60	5% or 4	N/A	Seated; BG = Big Gear
Hills	—	1–2x	1–2 min	2 min	42 x 14–16	40–60	3% or 3	N/A	Standing
Hills BG	—	1–2x	1–2 min	3 min	42 x 12–14	40–60	7% or 5	N/A	Seated
Hills*	—	1–2x	1–2 min	2 min	42 x 14–16	40–60	3% or 3	N/A	Sit and stand
Hills BG*	—	1–2x	1–2 min	3 min	42 x 12–14	40–60	10% or 7	N/A	Standing
Warm down	—	1x	5 min	—	42 x 18–21	85–95	0% or 1	LSD	Easy

EXTRA INFORMATION

Place training heart rates from page 42–43 in here.

* Remove these parts of your programme for a shorter/easier workout.

** Rest means easy active recovery pedalling (42 x 18–21).

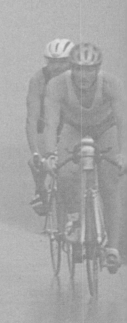

SPIN WORKOUT: Sub ③   **AIM:** High strength endurance   **TOTAL TIME:** 31–77 min
(1,2,3)

EXTRA INFORMATION

TRAIN TYPE	SET	REP	DURATION	REST**	GEAR	CADENCE	GRAD/RES	HEART RATE	EFFORT
Warm up	1-2x	1x	1 min	—	42 x 18-21	85-95	0% or 1	LSD	Easy
		1x	1 min	—	42 x 16-18	85-95	0% or 1	LSD	Easy
		1x	1 min	—	42 x 14-16	85-95	0% or 1	LSD	Easy
		1x	1 min	—	42 x 18-21	85-95	0% or 1	LSD	Easy
Hills	—	1x	2 min	1 min	42 x 14-16	40-60	3-5% or 2-4	N/A	Grunt
Hills BG	—	1x	2 min	2 min	42 x 12-14	40-60	7-10% or 5-7	N/A	Grunt; BG = Big Gear
Hills	—	1x	4 min	2 min	42 x 14-16	40-60	3-5% or 2-4	N/A	Grunt
Hills BG	—	1x	2 min	2 min	52 x 16-18	40-60	7-10% or 5-7	N/A	Grunt
Hills*	—	1x	4 min	2 min	42 x 14-16	40-60	3-5% or 2-4	N/A	Grunt
Hills BG*	—	1x	4 min	2 min	52 x 12-18	40-60	7-10% or 5-7	N/A	Grunt
Flat BG*	—	1x	10-20 min	—	52 x 14-18	40-60	0% or 1	N/A	Grunt; see pg 103
Warm down	—	1x	10-20 min	—	42 x 18-21	85-95	0% or 1	LSD	Easy

Place training heart rates from pages 42–43 in here.

3

* Remove these parts of your programme for a shorter/easier workout.
** Rest means easy active recovery pedalling (42 x 18-21).

PROGRAMME 3F — ADVANCED SPORT

SPIN WORKOUT: Sub ③ (1,2,3,4,6,7,8,9)

AIM: High strength endurance and speed maintenance

TOTAL TIME: 30–78 min

EXTRA INFORMATION

TRAIN TYPE	SET	REP	DURATION	REST**	GEAR	CADENCE	GRAD/RES	HEART RATE	EFFORT
Warm up	1–6x	1x	20 s	—	42 x 18-21	75-85	0% or 1	LSD	Easy
		1x	20 s	—	42 x 18-21	85-95	0% or 1	LSD	Easy
		1x	10 s	—	42 x 18-21	95-105	0% or 1	LSD	Easy
		1x	10 s	—	42 x 18-21	105-125	0% or 1	LSD	Easy
Power*	—	1x	10 s†	1 min	52 x 12-16	40→130	0% or 1	N/A	Explosive; see pg 128
Sprint (IS)*	—	1x	10–20 s†	1 min	52 x 14-18	85→120	0% or 1	N/A	Sprint top speed; see pg 123
AT*	—	1x	2 min	2 min	52 x 16-21	85-95	0% or 1	AT	Anaerobic threshold, hard
Hills	—	1x	2 min	2 min	42 x 14-16	40-60	3-5% or 2-4	N/A	Grunt
Hills BG	—	1x	2 min	—	52 x 16-18	40-60	7-10% or 5-7	N/A	Grunt; BG = Big Gear
Overspeed	—	1x	10 s†	3 min	42 x 18-21	105-135	0% or 1	N/A	Leg speed; see pg 134
Hills	—	1x	4 min	2 min	42 x 14-16	40-60	3-5% or 2-4	N/A	Grunt
Hills BG	—	1x	4 min	—	52 x 16-18	40-60	7-10% or 5-7	N/A	Grunt
Overspeed	—	1x	10 s†	3 min	42 x 18-21	105-135	0% or 1	N/A	Leg speed
Flat BG*	—	1x	10–20 min	—	52 x 14-18	60→80	0% or 1	N/A	Grunt; see pg 103
Warm down	—	1x	5–20 min	—	42 x 18-21	85-95	0% or 1	LSD	Easy

Place training heart rates from page 42–43 in here.

* Remove these parts of your programme for a shorter/easier workout.

** Rest means easy active recovery pedalling (42 x 18–21).

† Having completed the effort, pedal gently for the rest of the minute and begin the next part of the workout at the start of the next minute.

× Drafting, triathlon, duathlon, time trials, mountainbiking and multisport exclude.

4. Load/speed — 'transfer' training combining strength endurance and speed

Load/speed is the transition or conversion from strength training into speed training. This would occur from not at all to once or twice a week over a 2–8-week period (usually 2–4 weeks). It is emphasised at the end of Base.

SPECIFICS: Strength endurance moving to speed endurance. Riding on the flat in a big gear at low pedal cadence.

EFFORT: *During:* Medium effort (65–75 percent); medium muscular effort.

Between: Easy conversation pace (50–60 percent effort); easy muscular effort.

BIKE: Flat big gear.

Duration: Usually 10–20-minute intervals or longer; continuous duration.

During: On the flat in a big gear.
Gears: Medium/big gears; 52 or 53 x 12–16.
Cadence: 40–70 rpm or oscillating between 40 and 80 rpm.

Between: Easy riding.
Gears: Easy/small gears — small chainring (39 or 42 x 16–21).
Cadence: 85–95 rpm for time trialling, triathlon and duathlon; 95–105 rpm for road cycling and triathlon with legal drafting.

Training heart rate = During: N/A   Between:

(LSD: 60–75 percent HR^{max}).

See pages 42–43 for reference table.

SPIN WORKOUT: Sub ④
(1,4)

AIM: Strength endurance/
Speed

TOTAL TIME: 79 min
*39 min

EXTRA INFORMATION

TRAIN TYPE	DURATION	GEAR	CADENCE	EFFORT	HEART RATE	COMMENTS
Warm up	5 min	—	—	Easy	LSD	
Flat BG	1 min	↑↑	↓↓↓ 60	Grunt	N/A	BG = Big Gear
	1 min	↑↑	↓↓ 70	Grunt	N/A	
	1 min	↑↑	↓ 80	Grunt tempo	N/A	
Easy	5 min	—	—	Easy	LSD	
Flat BG	2 min	↑↑	↓↓↓ 60	Grunt	N/A	
	2 min	↑↑	↓↓ 70	Grunt	N/A	
	2 min	↑↑	↓ 80	Grunt tempo	N/A	
Easy	5 min	—	—	Easy	LSD	
Flat BG	2 min	↑↑	↓↓↓ 60	Grunt	N/A	
	2 min	↑↑	↓↓ 70	Grunt	N/A	
	1 min	↑↑	↓ 80	Grunt tempo	N/A	
	2 min	↑↑	↓↓↓ 60	Grunt	N/A	
	2 min	↑↑	↓↓ 70	Grunt	N/A	
	1 min	↑↑	↓ 80	Grunt tempo	N/A	
Easy*	5 min	—	—	Easy	LSD	
Flat BG*	6 min	↑↑	↓↓↓ 60	Grunt	N/A	
*	4 min	↑↑	↓↓ 70	Grunt	N/A	
*	2 min	↑↑	↓ 80	Grunt tempo	N/A	
Easy*	2 min	—	—	Easy	LSD	
Flat BG*	4 min	↑↑	↓↓ 70	Grunt	N/A	
*	6 min	↑↑	↓↓↓ 60	Grunt	N/A	
Easy*	5 min	—	—	Easy	LSD	
Flat BG*	2 min	↑↑	↓ 80	Grunt tempo	N/A	
*	2 min	↑↑	↓↓ 70	Grunt	N/A	
*	2 min	↑↑	↓↓↓ 60	Grunt	N/A	
Warm down	5 min	—	—	Easy	LSD	

Place training heart rates
from page 42–43 in here.

CODES	GEAR/RES	CADENCE
—	Usual/comfortable	Usual/comfortable
↑	A little harder (↑1–2 cogs)	A little higher (↑5 rpm)
↑↑	Moderately harder (↑2–3 cogs)	Moderately higher (↑10 rpm)
↑↑↑	Much harder (↑4–5 cogs)	Much higher (↑15⁺ rpm)
↓↓↓	Much easier (↓4–6 cogs)	Much lower (↓30 rpm)
↓↓	Moderately easier (↓2–4 cogs)	Moderately lower (↓20 rpm)
↓	A little easier (↓1–2 cogs)	A little lower (↓10 rpm)

*** Remove these parts
of your programme for
a shorter/easier
workout.**

PROGRAMME 4B

INTERMEDIATE SPORT

SPIN WORKOUT: Sub ④
(1,2,3,4)

AIM: Strength endurance/ Speed

TOTAL TIME: 79 min
*43 min

EXTRA INFORMATION

TRAIN TYPE	DURATION	GEAR	CADENCE	EFFORT	HEART RATE	COMMENTS
Warm up	5 min	—	—	Easy	LSD	
Hills	2 min	↑↑	↓↓	Grunt	N/A	
Easy	2 min	—	—	Easy	LSD	
Hills*	4 min	↑↑	↓↓	Grunt	N/A	
Easy*	2 min	—	—	Easy	LSD	
Hills BG	2 min	↑↑↑	↓↓↓	Grunt	N/A	BG = Big Gear
Easy	2 min	—	—	Easy	LSD	
Hills BG*	4 min	↑↑↑	↓↓↓	Grunt	N/A	
Easy*	2 min	—	—	Easy	LSD	
Flat BG	4 min	↑↑	↓↓↓ 60	Grunt	N/A	
	2 min	↑↑	↓↓ 70	Grunt	N/A	
	1 min	↑↑	↓ 80	Grunt tempo	N/A	
Easy	5 min	—	—	Easy	LSD	
Flat BG	2 min	↑↑	↓ 80	Grunt tempo	N/A	
	2 min	↑↑	↓↓ 70	Grunt	N/A	
	4 min	↑↑	↓↓↓ 60	Grunt	N/A	
Easy	5 min	—	—	Easy	LSD	
Hills*	2 min	↑↑	↓↓	Grunt	N/A	
Hills BG*	2 min	↑↑↑	↓↓↓	Grunt	N/A	
Easy*	2 min	—	—	Easy	LSD	
Flat BG*	4 min	↑↑	↓↓↓ 60	Grunt	N/A	
*	2 min	↑↑	↓↓ 70	Grunt	N/A	
*	1 min	↑↑	↓ 80	Grunt tempo	N/A	
Easy*	5 min	—	—	Easy	LSD	
Flat BG*	2 min	↑↑	↓↓↓ 60	Grunt	N/A	
*	2 min	↑↑	↓↓ 70	Grunt	N/A	
*	2 min	↑↑	↓ 80	Grunt tempo	N/A	
Warm down	5 min	—	—	Easy	LSD	

Place training heart rates from pages 42–43 in here.

* Remove these parts of your programme for a shorter/easier workout.

CODES	GEAR/RES	CADENCE
—	Usual/comfortable	Usual/comfortable
↑	A little harder (↑1–2 cogs)	A little higher (↑5 rpm)
↑↑	Moderately harder (↑2–3 cogs)	Moderately higher (↑10 rpm)
↑↑↑	Much harder (↑4–5 cogs)	Much higher (↑15⁺ rpm)
↓↓↓	Much easier (↓4–6 cogs)	Much lower (↓30 rpm)
↓↓	Moderately easier (↓2–4 cogs)	Moderately lower (↓20 rpm)
↓	A little easier (↓1–2 cogs)	A little lower (↓10 rpm)

4

SPIN WORKOUT: Sub ④   **AIM:** Strength endurance/Speed/   **TOTAL TIME:** 83 min
(1,2,3,4,5,6,7,8,9)   Speed maintenance   *38 min

EXTRA INFORMATION

TRAIN TYPE	DURATION	GEAR/RES	CADENCE	EFFORT	HEART RATE	COMMENTS
Warm up	5 min	—	—	Easy	LSD	
Overspeed*	10 s†	↓↓↓	↑↑↑	Leg speed	N/A	# §; see pg 134
Easy*	2 min	—	—	Easy	LSD	# §
Power*	10 s†	↑↑	↑↑	Explosive	N/A	#; see pg 128
Easy*	2 min	—	—	Easy	LSD	#
Sprint (IS)*	30 s†	↑↑	↑↑	Top speed	N/A	# §; see pg 123
Easy*	2 min	—	—	Easy	LSD	# §
AT*	3 min	—	—	Hard	AT	see pg 117
Easy*	3 min	—	—	Easy	LSD	
Tempo*	5 min	—	—	Tempo	UT	see pg 110
Easy*	5 min	—	—	Easy	LSD	
Hills	1–2 min	↑↑	↓↓	Grunt	N/A	
Easy	2 min	—	—	Easy	LSD	BG = Big Gear
Hills BG	1–2 min	↑↑↑	↓↓↓	Grunt	N/A	
Easy	2 min	—	—	Easy	LSD	
Flat BG	2–5 min	↑↑	↓↓ 60	Grunt	N/A	
Easy	2 min	—	—	Easy	LSD	
Flat BG	2–5 min	↑↑	↓↓ 70	Grunt	N/A	
Easy	2 min	—	—	Easy	LSD	
Flat BG	2–5 min	↑↑	↓↓ 80	Grunt tempo	N/A	
Easy	2 min	—	—	Easy	LSD	
Flat BG	2–5 min	↑↑	↓↓ 60	Grunt	N/A	
Easy	2 min	—	—	Easy	LSD	
Flat BG	2–5 min	↑↑	↓↓ 70	Grunt	N/A	
Easy	2 min	—	—	Easy	LSD	
Flat BG	2–5 min	↑↑	↓↓ 80	Grunt tempo	N/A	
Warm down	5 min	—	—	Easy	LSD	

 # Triathlon, duathlon and time trial exclude.

§ Drafting, tri/du/multi and mountainbiking exclude.

* Remove these parts of your programme for a shorter/easier workout.

† Having completed the effort, pedal gently for the rest of the minute and begin the next part of the workout at the start of the next minute.

Place training heart rates from pages 42–43 in here.

CODES	GEAR/RES	CADENCE
—	Usual/comfortable	Usual/comfortable
↑	A little harder (↑1–2 cogs)	A little higher (↑5 rpm)
↑↑	Moderately harder (↑2–3 cogs)	Moderately higher (↑10 rpm)
↑↑↑	Much harder (↑4–5 cogs)	Much higher (↑15+ rpm)
↓↓↓	Much easier (↓4–6 cogs)	Much lower (↓30 rpm)
↓↓	Moderately easier (↓2–4 cogs)	Moderately lower (↓20 rpm)
↓	A little easier (↓1–2 cogs)	A little lower (↓10 rpm)

PROGRAMME 4D   ADVANCED SPORT

SPIN WORKOUT: Sub ④ (1,4)

AIM: Strength endurance/Speed

TOTAL TIME: 33–92 min

EXTRA INFORMATION

TRAIN TYPE	SET	REP	DURATION	REST**	GEAR	CADENCE	GRAD/RES	HEART RATE	COMMENTS
Warm up	—	1x	5 min	—	42 x 18–21	85–95	0% or 1	LSD	Easy
Flat BG*	—	1x	5–10 min	—	52 x 14–18	40–50	0% or 1	N/A	Grunt; BG = Big Gear
Easy*	—	1x	5 min	—	42 x 16–18	85–95	0% or 1	LSD	Easy
Flat BG*	—	1x	5–10 min	—	52 x 14–18	50–60	0% or 1	N/A	Grunt
Easy*	—	1x	5 min	—	42 x 16–18	85–95	0% or 1	LSD	Easy
Flat BG	—	1x	5–10 min	—	52 x 14–18	60–70	0% or 1	N/A	Grunt
Easy	—	1x	5 min	—	42 x 16–18	85–95	0% or 1	LSD	Easy
Flat BG	—	1x	5–10 min	—	52 x 14–18	70–80	0% or 1	N/A	Grunt/tempo
Easy	—	1x	5 min	—	42 x 16–18	85–95	0% or 1	LSD	Easy
Flat BG	—	1x	3 min	—	52 x 14–18	80+	0% or 1	N/A	Grunt/tempo
Easy*	—	1x	5 min	—	42 x 16–18	85–95	0% or 1	LSD	Easy
BG*	—	3x	1 min	—	52 x 12–16	40–60	0% or 1	N/A	Tech; see pg 57
Little gear	—		1 min	1 min	42 x 18–21	100–125	0% or 1		
Warm down	—	1x	5–10 min	—	42 x 18–21	85–95	0% or 1	LSD	Easy

Place training heart rates from pages 42–43 in here.

* Remove these parts of your programme for a shorter/easier workout.
** Rest means easy active recovery pedalling (42 x 18–21).

SPIN WORKOUT: Sub ④ (1,2,3,4,5)   **AIM:** Strength endurance/Speed   **TOTAL TIME:** 36–79 min

EXTRA INFORMATION

TRAIN TYPE	SET	REP	DURATION	REST**	GEAR	CADENCE	GRAD/RES	HEART RATE	COMMENTS
Warm up	—	1x	1 min	—	42 x 18-21	85-95	0% or 1	LSD	Easy
	—	1x	1 min	—	42 x 16-18	85-95	0% or 1	LSD	Easy
	—	1x	1 min	—	42 x 14-16	85-95	0% or 1	LSD	Easy
	—	1x	1 min	—	42 x 18-21	85-95	0% or 1	LSD	Easy
Flat BG	—	1x	10 min	—	52 x 14-18	1 min @ 60 / 1 min @ 70 / 1 min @ 80	0% or 1	N/A	Grunt; BG = Big Gear
Over speed	—	1x	30 s†	—	42 x 18-21	85 → 140	0% or 1	N/A	Leg speed; see pg 134
Easy	—	1x	5 min	—	42 x 14-16	85-95	0% or 1	LSD	Easy
Flat BG	—	1x	10 min	—	52 x 14-18	1 min @ 60 / 1 min @ 70 / 1 min @ 80	0% or 1	N/A	Grunt
Overspeed	—	1x	30 s†	—	42 x 18-21	85 → 140	0% or 1	N/A	Leg speed
Easy*	—	1x	5 min	—	42 x 14-16	85-95	0% or 1	LSD	Easy
Hills*	—	1-3x	2 min	1 min	42 x 14-16	40-60	3% or 2	N/A	Grunt
Hills BG*	—	1-3x	2 min	1 min	42 x 12-15	40-60	5-7% or 3-5	N/A	Grunt
Flat BG*	—	1x	10-20 min	—	52 x 14-18	2 min @ 60 / 2 min @ 70 / 2 min @ 80	0% or 1	N/A	Grunt
Warm down	—	1x	5 min	—	42 x 18-21	85-95	0% or 1	LSD	Easy

Place training heart rates from pages 42–43 in here.

* Remove these parts of your programme for a shorter/easier workout.

** Rest means easy active recovery pedalling (42 x 18–21).

† Having completed the effort, pedal gently for the rest of the minute and begin the next part of the workout at the start of the next minute.

SPIN WORKOUT: Sub ④ (1,2,3,4,6,7,8,9)

AIM: Strength endurance/Speed /Speed maintenance

TOTAL TIME: 24–54 min

EXTRA INFORMATION

TRAIN TYPE	SET	REP	DURATION	REST**	GEAR	CADENCE	GRAD/RES	HEART RATE	COMMENTS
Warm up	1–6x	1x	20 s	—	42 x 18–21	75–85	0% or 1	LSD	Easy
		1x	20 s	—	42 x 18–21	85–95	0% or 1	LSD	Easy
		1x	10 s	—	42 x 18–21	95–105	0% or 1	LSD	Easy
		1x	10 s	—	42 x 18–21	105–125	0% or 1	LSD	Easy
Overspeed*	—	1x	10 s†	1 min	42 x 18–21	105→140	0% or 1	N/A	Leg speed # §; see pg 134
Power*	—	1x	10 s†	1 min	52 x 12–16	40→130	0% or 1	N/A	Explosive #; see pg 128
Sprint (IS)*	—	1x	30 s†	1 min	52 x 14–18	85→120	0% or 1	N/A	Sprint top speed # §; see pg 123
AT*	—	1x	2 min	2 min	52 x 16–21	85–95	0% or 1	AT	Hard; see pg 117
Hills	—	1x	2 min	—	42 x 14–16	40–60	3–5% or 2–4	N/A	Grunt
Flat BG	—	1x	5–10 min	—	52 x 14–18	1 min @ 60 / 1 min @ 70 / 1 min @ 80	0% or 1	N/A	Grunt tempo
Hills	—	1x	2 min	—	42 x 14–16	40–60	3–5% or 2–4	N/A	Grunt
Flat BG	—	1x	5–10 min	—	52 x 14–18	1 min @ 60 / 1 min @ 70 / 1 min @ 80	0% or 1	N/A	Grunt tempo
Hills	—	1x	2 min	—	42 x 14–16	40–60	3–5% or 2–4	N/A	Grunt
Hills BG	—	1x	2 min	—	52 x 16–18	40–60	5–7% or 4–6	N/A	Grunt
Warm down	—	1x	5–10 min	—	42 x 18–21	85–95	0% or 1	LSD	Easy

Place training heart rates from pages 42–43 in here.

* Remove these parts of your programme for a shorter/easier workout.
** Rest means easy active recovery pedalling (42 x 18–21).
† Having completed the effort, pedal gently for the rest of the minute and begin the next part of the workout at the start of the next minute.

Triathlon, duathlon and time trial exclude.

§ Drafting, tri/du/multi and mountainbiking exclude.

4

5. Low-speed work — up-tempo training

Low-speed work is the beginning of conditioning for speed. This form of speed work is at tempo (feeling fast but strong and in control); it is about 10 beats below anaerobic threshold. This would occur once or twice a week and would be gradually phased in over a period of 2–4 weeks (usually 2 weeks). The emphasis is at the end of Base for races under 4 hours and at the start of Speed for races over 4 hours.

SPECIFICS: Up-tempo — long intervals at tempo pace (Ironman, tour race pace); should feel fast and strong. Riding at tempo pace in a normal gear.

EFFORT: *During:* Moderately difficult to converse (70–75 percent effort); medium muscular effort.

Between: Easy conversation pace (50–60 percent effort); easy muscular effort.

BIKE: Up-tempo — tempo riding — not race pace and not cruising; you should feel fast, strong, comfortable and in control. The pace is equivalent to maximum 3-hour race pace (i.e. the hardest you could go for 3 hours, no harder). Harder is not better, just the wrong intensity (maximum 3-hour pace, not maximum pace that you can do the interval).

Duration: Usually 10–20-minute intervals.

During: Tempo intervals.
Gears: Medium gears; 39 or 42 x 12–16 for most people; 52 or 53 x 14–18 for 'rock stars'.
Cadence: 85–95 rpm for time trialling, triathlon and duathlon; 95–105 rpm for road cycling and triathlon with legal drafting.

Between: Easy riding.
Gears: Easy/small gears — small chainring (39 or 42 x 16–21).
Cadence: 85–95 rpm for time trialling, triathlon and duathlon; 95–105 rpm for road cycling and triathlon with legal drafting.

Training heart rate = During: ☐ (UT) for intervals

Between: ☐ (LSD: 60–75 percent HR^{max}).
See pages 42–43 for reference table.

SPIN WORKOUT: Sub ⑤
(1,5)

AIM: Low speedwork

TOTAL TIME: 44–52 min
or 35–45 min

EXTRA INFORMATION

TRAIN TYPE	DURATION*	GEAR/RES	CADENCE	EFFORT	HEART RATE	COMMENTS
Warm up	5 min	—	—	Easy	LSD	
Up tempo	1 min	—	—	Tempo	UT	
Easy	2 min	—	—	Easy	LSD	
Up tempo	2 min	—	—	Tempo	UT	
Easy	2 min	—	—	Easy	LSD	
Up tempo	4 min	—	—	Tempo	UT	
Easy	4→1 min	—	—	Easy	LSD	
Up tempo	6 min	—	—	Tempo	UT	
Easy	6→1 min	—	—	Easy	LSD	
Up tempo	10 min	—	—	Tempo	UT	
Warm down	10 min	—	—	Easy	LSD	
OR						
Warm up	5 min	—	—	Easy	LSD	
Up tempo	20–30 min	—	—	Tempo	UT	
Warm down	10 min	—	—	Easy	LSD	

Place training heart rates
from pages 42–43 in here.

*Over a period of time drop or increase the workout or recovery time so 1→3 means increase from 1 to 3 min over a period of weeks and 3→1 means decrease in the same way. Always start with the recovery at the longest duration and the effort at the shortest duration.

CODES	GEAR/RES	CADENCE
—	Usual/comfortable	Usual/comfortable
↑	A little harder (↑1–2 cogs)	A little higher (↑5 rpm)
↑↑	Moderately harder (↑2–3 cogs)	Moderately higher (↑10 rpm)
↑↑↑	Much harder (↑4–5 cogs)	Much higher (↑15+ rpm)
↓↓↓	Much easier (↓4–6 cogs)	Much lower (↓30 rpm)
↓↓	Moderately easier (↓2–4 cogs)	Moderately lower (↓20 rpm)
↓	A little easier (↓1–2 cogs)	A little lower (↓10 rpm)

SPIN WORKOUT: Sub ⑤ (1,4,5) **AIM:** Low speedwork **TOTAL TIME:** 69 min *37 min

EXTRA INFORMATION

TRAIN TYPE	DURATION	GEAR/RES	CADENCE	EFFORT	HEART RATE	COMMENTS
Warm up	5 min	—	—	Easy	LSD	
Up tempo	2 min	—	—	Tempo	UT	
Easy	2 min	—	—	Easy	LSD	
Up tempo	4 min	—	—	Tempo	UT	
Easy	2 min	—	—	Easy	LSD	
Flat BG*	10 min	↑↑	↓↓	Grunt	N/A	
Easy*	4 min	—	—	Easy	LSD	
Hills BG*	4 min	↑↑↑	↓↓↓	Grunt	N/A	
Easy*	4 min	—	—	Easy	LSD	
Hills	2 min	↑↑	↓↓	Grunt	N/A	
Easy	2 min	—	—	Easy	LSD	
Up tempo	2 min	—	—	Tempo	UT	
Easy	2 min	—	—	Easy	LSD	
Up tempo	4 min	—	—	Tempo	UT	
Easy*	4 min	—	—	Easy	LSD	
Up tempo*	6 min	—	—	Tempo	UT	
Warm down	10 min	—	—	Easy	LSD	

* Remove these parts of your programme for a shorter/easier workout.

Place training heart rates from pages 42–43 in here.

CODES	GEAR/RES	CADENCE
—	Usual/comfortable	Usual/comfortable
↑	A little harder (↑1–2 cogs)	A little higher (↑5 rpm)
↑↑	Moderately harder (↑2–3 cogs)	Moderately higher (↑10 rpm)
↑↑↑	Much harder (↑4–5 cogs)	Much higher (↑15+ rpm)
↓↓↓	Much easier (↓4–6 cogs)	Much lower (↓30 rpm)
↓↓	Moderately easier (↓2–4 cogs)	Moderately lower (↓20 rpm)
↓	A little easier (↓1–2 cogs)	A little lower (↓10 rpm)

SPIN WORKOUT: Sub ⑤   **AIM:** Low speedwork/   **TOTAL TIME:** 65 min
(1,5,6,7,8,9)   Speed maintenance   *40 min

EXTRA INFORMATION

TRAIN TYPE	DURATION	GEAR/RES	CADENCE	EFFORT	HEART RATE	COMMENTS
Warm up	5 min	—	—	Easy	LSD	
Overspeed*	10 s†	↓↓↓	↑↑↑	Leg speed	N/A	# §; see pg 134
Easy*	2 min	—	—	Easy	LSD	# §
Up tempo	2 min	—	—	Tempo	UT	
Easy	2 min	—	—	Easy	LSD	
Power*	10 s†	↑↑	↑↑	Explosive	N/A	#; see pg 128
Easy*	2 min	—	—	Easy	LSD	#
Up tempo	4 min	—	—	Tempo	UT	
Easy	4 min	—	—	Easy	LSD	
Sprint (IS)*	20–30 s†	↑↑	↑↑	Sprint	N/A	Top speed # §; see pg 123
Easy*	4 min	—	—	Easy	LSD	# §;
Up tempo	2–6 min	—	—	Tempo	UT	
Easy	4 min	—	—	Easy	LSD	
AT	1–3 min	—	—	Hard	AT	see pg 117
Easy	4 min	—	—	Easy	LSD	
Up tempo	2–10 min	—	—	Tempo	UT	
Warm down	10 min	—	—	Easy	LSD	

> Place training heart rates from pages 42–43 in here.

 # Triathlon, duathlon and time trial exclude.

§ Drafting, tri/du/multi and mountainbiking exclude.

* Remove these parts of your programme for a shorter/easier workout.

† Having completed the effort, pedal gently for the rest of the minute and begin the next part of the workout at the start of the next minute.

CODES	GEAR/RES	CADENCE
—	Usual/comfortable	Usual/comfortable
↑	A little harder (↑1–2 cogs)	A little higher (↑5 rpm)
↑↑	Moderately harder (↑2–3 cogs)	Moderately higher (↑10 rpm)
↑↑↑	Much harder (↑4–5 cogs)	Much higher (↑15⁺ rpm)
↓↓↓	Much easier (↓4–6 cogs)	Much lower (↓30 rpm)
↓↓	Moderately easier (↓2–4 cogs)	Moderately lower (↓20 rpm)
↓	A little easier (↓1–2 cogs)	A little lower (↓10 rpm)

SPIN WORKOUT: Sub ⑤ (1,5)   **AIM:** Low speedwork   **TOTAL TIME:** 24–61 min

EXTRA INFORMATION

TRAIN TYPE	SET	REP	DURATION	REST	GEAR	CADENCE	GRAD/RES	HEART RATE	COMMENTS
Warm up	—	1x	5 min	—	42 x 18–21	85–95	0% or 1	LSD	Easy
Up tempo	—	1x	1 min	—	42 x 12–16	85–95	0% or 1	UT	Tempo
Easy	—	1x	1 min	—	42 x 16–18	85–95	0% or 1	LSD	Easy
Up tempo	—	1x	2 min	—	42 x 12–16	85–95	0% or 1	UT	Tempo
Easy	—	1x	2 min	—	42 x 16–18	85–95	0% or 1	LSD	Easy
Up tempo	—	1x	4 min	—	42 x 12–16	85–95	0% or 1	UT	Tempo
Easy	—	1x	4 min	—	42 x 16–18	85–95	0% or 1	LSD	Easy
Up tempo*	—	1x	6 min	—	42 x 12–16	85–95	0% or 1	UT	Tempo
Easy*	—	1x	6 min	—	42 x 16–18	85–95	0% or 1	LSD	Easy
Up tempo*	—	1x	10 min	—	42 x 12–16	85–95	0% or 1	UT	Tempo
Warm down	—	1x	5–20 min	—	42 x 18–21	85–95	0% or 1	LSD	Easy

Place training heart rates from pages 42–43 in here.

* Remove these parts of your programme for a shorter/easier workout.

SPIN WORKOUT: Sub (5)
(1,2,4,5)

AIM: Low speedwork

TOTAL TIME: 30–71 min

TRAIN TYPE	SET	REP	DURATION	REST		GEAR	CADENCE	GRAD/RES	HEART RATE	COMMENTS
Warm up	1–6x	1x	20 s	—		42 x 18–21	75–85	0% or 1	LSD	Easy
		1x	20 s	—		42 x 18–21	85–95	0% or 1	LSD	Easy
		1x	10 s	—		42 x 18–21	95–105	0% or 1	LSD	Easy
		1x	10 s	—		42 x 18–21	105–125	0% or 1	LSD	Easy
Up tempo	—	1x	2 min	—		42 x 12–16	85–95	0% or 1	LT	Tempo
Easy	—	1x	2 min	—		42 x 16–18	85–95	0% or 1	LSD	Easy
Up tempo	—	1x	4 min	—		42 x 12–16	85–95	0% or 1	LT	Tempo
Hills	—	1x	2 min	—		42 x 14–16	40–60	3–5% or 2–4	N/A	Grunt
Easy	—	1x	5 min	—		42 x 16–18	85–95	0% or 1	LSD	Easy
Flat BG*	—	1x	10 min	—		52 x 14–18	40–60	0% or 1	N/A	Grunt
Up tempo	—	1x	2–10 min	—		42 x 12–16	85–95	0% or 1	LT	Tempo
Easy	—	1x	5 min	—		42 x 16–18	85–95	0% or 1	LSD	Easy
Up tempo	—	1x	2–10 min	—		42 x 12–16	85–95	0% or 1	LT	Tempo
Flat BG*	—	1x	10 min	—		52 x 14–18	70–80	0% or 1	N/A	Grunt tempo
Warm down	—	1x	5 min	—		42 x 18–21	85–95	0% or 1	LSD	Easy

EXTRA INFORMATION

Place training heart rates from pages 42–43 in here.

* **Remove these parts of your programme for a shorter/easier workout.**

AIM: Low speedwork   **TOTAL TIME:** 34–59 min

SPIN WORKOUT: Sub ⑤
(1,2,3,4,5,9)

EXTRA INFORMATION

TRAIN TYPE	SET	REP	DURATION	REST**	GEAR	CADENCE	GRAD/RES	HEART RATE	COMMENTS
Warm up	1–2x	⎧1x	1 min	—	42 x 18–21	85–95	0% or 1	LSD	Easy
		1x	1 min	—	42 x 16–18	85–95	0% or 1	LSD	Easy
		1x	1 min	—	42 x 14–16	85–95	0% or 1	LSD	Easy
		⎩1x	1 min	—	42 x 18–21	85–95	0% or 1	LSD	Easy
Overspeed*	—	1x	10 s†	1 min	42 x 18–21	85→140	0% or 1	N/A	Leg speed
Long Sp (ES)*	—	1x	1 min	2 min	52 x 14–16	85→120	0% or 1	N/A	Extended sprint
Up tempo	—	1x	2 min	—	42 x 12–16	85–95	0% or 1	UT	Up tempo
Easy	—	1x	2 min	—	42 x 16–18	85–95	0% or 1	LSD	Easy
Up tempo	—	1x	4 min	—	42 x 12–16	85–95	0% or 1	UT	Tempo
Easy	—	1x	4 min	—	42 x 16–18	85–95	0% or 1	LSD	Easy
Up tempo	—	1x	4–10 min	—	42 x 12–16	85–95	0% or 1	UT	Up tempo
Hills	—	1x	2 min	—	42 x 14–16	40–60	3–5% or 2–4	N/A	Grunt
Hills BG	—	1x	2 min	—	42 x 12–15	40–60	5–7% or 4–6	N/A	Grunt
Flat BG	—	1x	5–10 min	—	52 x 14–18	40–70	0% or 1	N/A	Grunt
Warm down	—	1x*	5–10 min	—	42 x 18–21	85–95	0% or 1	LSD	Easy

Place training heart rates from pages 42–43 in here.

* **Remove these parts of your programme for a shorter/easier workout.**

** **Rest means easy active recovery pedalling (42 x 18–21).**

† **Having completed the effort, pedal gently for the rest of the minute and begin the next part of the workout at the start of the next minute.**

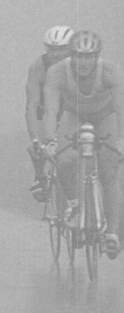

6. High-speed work — anaerobic threshold training

High-speed work is used to boost your anaerobic threshold or maximum steady-state pace (40-km time trial pace). It involves short, intense intervals, and you should feel as if you are 'hammering'. This subphase lasts over a 2–8-week period (usually 1–4 weeks). It is emphasised at the start of Speed training for races less than 4 hours and in the middle of Speed for races over 4 hours.

SPECIFICS: Anaerobic threshold training — short intervals generally of 5–8 minutes (40-km bike time-trial pace); you should feel like you are hammering. Riding at anaerobic threshold pace in a normal gear.

EFFORT: *During:* Difficult to converse (75–85 percent effort); medium muscular effort.

Between: Easy conversation pace (50–60 percent effort); easy muscular effort.

BIKE: Anaerobic threshold — riding at time-trial or race pace (average). You should feel you are on the edge between being in control and being out of control and sprinting, and be just on the verge of puffing hard. The pace is equivalent to maximum 20-minute to 1-hour race pace (i.e. the hardest you could go for 20 minutes to 1 hour, no harder). Harder is not better, just the wrong intensity (maximum 1-hour pace, not maximum pace that you can do the interval). This is hard but not hell!

Duration: Usually 1–4-minute intervals.

During: Anaerobic threshold (race pace) intervals.
Gears: Medium/big gears; 39 or 42 x 12–16 for most people; 52 or 53 x 14–18 for 'rock stars'.
Cadence: 85–95 rpm for time trialling, triathlon and duathlon; 95–105 rpm for road cycling and triathlon with legal drafting.

Between: Easy riding.
Gears: Easy/small gears — small chainring (39 or 42 x 16–21).
Cadence: 85–95 rpm for time trialling, triathlon and duathlon; 95–105 rpm for road cycling and triathlon with legal drafting.

Training heart rate = During: ☐ (AT) for intervals

Between: ☐ (LSD: 60–75 percent HR^{max}).
See pages 42–43 for reference table.

SPIN WORKOUT: Sub ⑥ **AIM:** High speedwork **TOTAL TIME:** 30–60 min
(1,6)

EXTRA INFORMATION

TRAIN TYPE	DURATION*	GEAR	CADENCE	EFFORT	HEART RATE	COMMENTS
Warm up	5 min	—	—	Easy	LSD	
AT	1→3 min	—	—	Hard	AT	
Easy	3→1 min	—	—	Easy	LSD	
AT	1→3 min	—	—	Hard	AT	
Easy	3→1 min	—	—	Easy	LSD	
AT	1→3 min	—	—	Hard	AT	
Easy	3→1 min	—	—	Easy	LSD	
AT	1→3 min	—	—	Hard	AT	
Easy	3→1 min	—	—	Easy	LSD	
AT	1→3 min	—	—	Hard	AT	
Easy	3→1 min	—	—	Easy	LSD	
AT	1→3 min	—	—	Hard	AT	
Easy	3→1 min	—	—	Easy	LSD	
AT	1→3 min	—	—	Hard	AT	
Easy	3→1 min	—	—	Easy	LSD	
AT	1→3 min	—	—	Hard	AT	
Warm down	10 min	—	—	Easy	LSD	

Place training heart rates from pages 42–43 in here.

* Over a period of time drop or increase the workout or recovery time so 1→3 means increase from 1 to 3 min over a period of weeks and 3→1 means decrease in the same way. Always start with the recovery at the longest duration and the effort at the shortest duration.

CODES	GEAR/RES	CADENCE
—	Usual/comfortable	Usual/comfortable
↑	A little harder (↑1–2 cogs)	A little higher (↑5 rpm)
↑↑	Moderately harder (↑2–3 cogs)	Moderately higher (↑10 rpm)
↑↑↑	Much harder (↑4–5 cogs)	Much higher (↑15+ rpm)
↓↓↓	Much easier (↓4–6 cogs)	Much lower (↓30 rpm)
↓↓	Moderately easier (↓2–4 cogs)	Moderately lower (↓20 rpm)
↓	A little easier (↓1–2 cogs)	A little lower (↓10 rpm)

SPIN WORKOUT: Sub ⑥
(1,5,6)

AIM: High speedwork

TOTAL TIME: 38–74 min

EXTRA INFORMATION

TRAIN TYPE	DURATION*	GEAR	CADENCE	EFFORT	HEART RATE	COMMENTS
Warm up	5 min	—	—	Easy	LSD	
Up tempo	2→5 min	—	—	Tempo	UT	
Easy	5→1 min	—	—	Easy	LSD	
AT	2→4 min	—	—	Hard	AT	
Easy	5→1 min	—	—	Easy	LSD	
AT	2→4 min	—	—	Hard	AT	
Easy	5→1 min	—	—	Easy	LSD	
AT	4→6 min	—	—	Hard	AT	
Easy	5→1 min	—	—	Easy	LSD	
Up tempo	2→5 min	—	—	Tempo	UT	
Easy	5→1 min	—	—	Easy	LSD	
Up tempo	6–10 min	—	—	Tempo	UT	
Warm down	10 min	—	—	Easy	LSD	

* Over a period of time drop or increase the workout or recovery time so 1→3 means increase from 1 to 3 min over a period of weeks and 3→1 means decrease in the same way. Always start with the recovery at the longest duration and the effort at the shortest duration.

Place training heart rates from pages 42–43 in here.

CODES	GEAR/RES	CADENCE
—	Usual/comfortable	Usual/comfortable
↑	A little harder (↑1–2 cogs)	A little higher (↑5 rpm)
↑↑	Moderately harder (↑2–3 cogs)	Moderately higher (↑10 rpm)
↑↑↑	Much harder (↑4–5 cogs)	Much higher (↑15+ rpm)
↓↓↓	Much easier (↓4–6 cogs)	Much lower (↓30 rpm)
↓↓	Moderately easier (↓2–4 cogs)	Moderately lower (↓20 rpm)
↓	A little easier (↓1–2 cogs)	A little lower (↓10 rpm)

SPIN WORKOUT: Sub ⑥   **AIM:** Speedwork and Speed/   **TOTAL TIME:** 38–77 min
(1,2,3,4,6,7,8,9)   Strength endurance maintenance

EXTRA INFORMATION

TRAIN TYPE	DURATION	GEAR	CADENCE	EFFORT	HEART RATE	COMMENTS
Warm up	5 min	—	—	Easy	LSD	
Overspeed*	10 s†	↓↓↓	↑↑↑	Leg speed	N/A	# §; see pg 134
Easy*	2 min	—	—	Easy	LSD	# §
Power*	10 s†	↑↑	↑↑	Explosive	N/A	#; see pg 128
Easy*	2 min	—	—	Easy	LSD	#
Sprint (IS)*	20–30 s†	↑↑	↑	Sprint	N/A	Top speed # §; see pg 123
Easy*	2 min	—	—	Easy	LSD	# §
AT	1–3 min	—	—	Hard	AT	
Easy	5 min	—	—	Easy	LSD	
AT	2–5 min	—	—	Hard	AT	
Easy	5 min	—	—	Easy	LSD	
AT*	3–5 min	—	—	Hard	AT	
Easy*	5 min	—	—	Easy	LSD	
Hills	2 min	↑↑	↓↓	Grunt	N/A	
Easy	3 min	—	—	Easy	LSD	
Hills*	2 min	↑↑	↓↓	Grunt	N/A	
Easy*	3 min	—	—	Easy	LSD	
Hills BG	2 min	↑↑↑	↓↓↓	Grunt	N/A	
Easy	3 min	—	—	Easy	LSD	
Flat BG	5–10 min	↑↑	↓↓	Grunt	N/A	
Warm down	5–10 min	—	—	Easy	LSD	

Place training heart rates from pages 42–43 in here.

* Remove these parts of your programme for a shorter/easier workout.

† Having completed the effort, pedal gently for the rest of the minute and begin the next part of the workout at the start of the next minute.

CODES	GEAR/RES	CADENCE
—	Usual/comfortable	Usual/comfortable
↑	A little harder (↑1–2 cogs)	A little higher (↑5 rpm)
↑↑	Moderately harder (↑2–3 cogs)	Moderately higher (↑10 rpm)
↑↑↑	Much harder (↑4–5 cogs)	Much higher (↑15+ rpm)
↓↓↓	Much easier (↓4–6 cogs)	Much lower (↓30 rpm)
↓↓	Moderately easier (↓2–4 cogs)	Moderately lower (↓20 rpm)
↓	A little easier (↓1–2 cogs)	A little lower (↓10 rpm)

 # Triathlon, duathlon and time trial exclude.

§ Drafting, tri/du/multi and mountainbiking exclude.

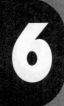

SPIN WORKOUT: Sub ⑥ (1,2,3,4,6)

AIM: High speedwork and Strength endurance maintenance

TOTAL TIME: 38–65 min

EXTRA INFORMATION

TRAIN TYPE	SET	REP	DURATION	REST**	GEAR	CADENCE	GRAD/RES	HEART RATE	COMMENTS
Warm up	—	1x	5 min	—	42 x 18-21	85-95	0% or 1	LSD	Easy
AT	—	1x	30 s'	1 min	52 x 16-18	85-95	0% or 1	AT	Hard
	—	1x	1 min	1 min	52 x 16-18	85-95	0% or 1	AT	Hard
*	—	1x	3 min	1 min	52 x 16-18	85-95	0% or 1	AT	Hard
*	—	1x	5 min	1 min	52 x 16-18	85-95	0% or 1	AT	Hard
*	—	1x	3 min	1 min	52 x 14-16	85-95	0% or 1	AT	Hard
*	—	1x	1 min	1 min	52 x 14-16	85-95	0% or 1	AT	Hard
	—	1x	30 s'	1 min	52 x 12-14	85-95	0% or 1	AT	Hard
Easy	—	1x	5-10 min	2 min	42 x 16-18	85-95	0% or 1	LSD	Easy
Hills	—	1x	2 min	2 min	42 x 14-16	40-60	3-5% or 2-4	N/A	Grunt
Hills BG	—	1x	2 min	2 min	42 x 12-15	40-60	5-7% or 4-6	N/A	Grunt
Flat BG	—	1x	5-10 min	—	52 x 14-18	2 @ 60 1 @ 70 1 @ 80	0% or 1	N/A	Grunt
Warm down	—	1x	5-10 min	—	42 x 18-21	85-95	0% or 1	LSD	Easy

Place training heart rates from pages 42–43 in here.

* Remove these parts of your programme for a shorter/easier workout.

** Rest means easy active recovery pedalling (42 x 18-21).

† Having completed the effort, pedal gently for the rest of the minute and begin the next part of the workout at the start of the next minute.

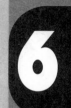

PROGRAMME 6E ADVANCED SPORT

SPIN WORKOUT: Sub ⑥ (1,2,5,6) **AIM:** High and low speedwork **TOTAL TIME:** 54–73 min

TRAIN TYPE	SET	REP	DURATION	REST*	GEAR	CADENCE	GRAD/RES	HEART RATE	COMMENTS
Warm up	—	1x	5 min	—	42 x 18–21	85–95	0% or 1	LSD	Easy
Up tempo	—	1x	3 min	3 min	42 x 12–16	85–95	0% or 1	UT	Tempo
AT	—	1x	2 min	2 min	52 x 14–16	85–95	0% or 1	AT	Hard
Up tempo	—	1x	5 min	5 min	42 x 12–16	85–95	0% or 1	UT	Tempo
AT	—	1x	3 min	3 min	52 x 14–16	85–95	0% or 1	AT	Hard
		1–3x	2–4 min	2 min	52 x 14–16	85–95	0% or 1	AT	Hard
Up tempo	—	1x	5–10 min	5 min	42 x 12–16	85–95	0% or 1	UT	Tempo
Hills	—	1x	2 min	2 min	42 x 14–16	40–60	3–5% or 2–4	N/A	Grunt
Warm down	—	1x	5 min	—	42 x 18–21	85–95	0% or 1	LSD	Easy

EXTRA INFORMATION

Place training heart rates from pages 42–43 in here.

* Rest means easy active recovery pedalling (42 x 18–21).

7. Sprints (extensive and intensive) — low and high anaerobic speed

Sprints involve, not surprisingly, sprinting. They can be broken down into two types: extensive and intensive sprints. Extensive sprints are long sprints (anaerobic lactic) lasting between 45 seconds and 4 minutes. They improve speed endurance. Intensive sprints are short sprints (anaerobic alactic) lasting between 10 seconds and 1 minute. They improve top speed.

Sprint training occurs once or twice a week over a 1–4-week period (usually 2 weeks). It is emphasised in the middle to end of Speed training.

SPECIFICS: Extensive sprints (long sprints) last 45 seconds to 4 minutes.

Intensive sprints (short sprints) last 10 seconds to 1 minute.

Sprinting at normal pace in a normal gear.

EFFORT: *During:* Very difficult to converse (90–100 percent effort); high muscular effort.

Between: Easy conversation pace (50–60 percent effort); easy muscular effort.

BIKE: Extensive sprint (long sprint) — nearly full effort extended sprint, like launching a lone attack 1–2 km from the finish of a road race or bridging a gap (like a pursuit). Welcome to hell!

Intensive sprint (short sprint) — full effort sprint that you might do at the finish of a road race. There are four variations:

Flat: 100–300 m on the flat; Crest: 30 m up and 20 m over the top; Uphill: 50 m up; Varied recovery: sprint then varied 10–30-second recovery and sprint again.

Don't get bogged down or buried by the gear; pull out before this happens.

Duration: Extensive sprint — 30 seconds to 4 minutes.

Intensive sprint — 10 to 30 seconds.

During: Long and short sprint reps.

Gears: Big gears; 52 or 53 x 12–18.

Cadence: Approx. 85–160 rpm.

Between: Easy riding.

Gears: Easy/small gears — small chainring; 39 or 42 x 16–21.

Cadence: 85–95 rpm for time trialling, triathlon and duathlon; 95–105 rpm for road cycling and triathlon with legal drafting.

Training heart rate = During: N/A   Between: ☐

(LSD: 60–75 percent HR^{max}).

See pages 42–43 for reference table.

NOTE: Intensive sprints can be broken into uphill, crest and flat. The uphill sprints are performed at a higher resistance (bigger gear, higher gradient) than the flat sprints (watch for wheel slippage on the trainer).

SPIN WORKOUT: Sub ⑦   **AIM:** Sprint (anaerobic) speed   **TOTAL TIME:** 81 min
(1,7,9)   *33 min

EXTRA INFORMATION

TRAIN TYPE	DURATION**	GEAR/RES	CADENCE	EFFORT	HEARTRATE	COMMENTS
Warm up	5–10 min	—	—	Easy	LSD	
Overspeed	10 s†	↓↓↓	↑↑↑	Leg speed	N/A	see pg 134
Easy	2 min	—	—	Easy	LSD	
Overspeed*	10 s†	↓↓↓	↑↑↑	Leg speed	N/A	
Easy*	2 min	—	—	Easy	LSD	
Flat sprint*	20–30 s†	↑	↑	Sprint	N/A	Top speed
Easy*	5→3 min	—	—	Easy	LSD	
Crest sprint*	20–30 s†	↑ then —	↑	Sprint	N/A	Strength
Easy*	5→3 min	—	—	Easy	LSD	
Uphill sprint	20–30 s†	↑↑	↑	Sprint	N/A	Strength
Easy	5→3 min	—	—	Easy	LSD	
Flat sprint*	20–30 s†	↑	↑	Sprint	N/A	Top speed
Easy*	5 min	—	—	Easy	LSD	
Crest sprint*	20–30 s†	↑ then —	↑	Sprint	N/A	Strength
Easy*	5→3 min	—	—	Easy	LSD	
Uphill sprint	20–30 s†	↑↑	↑	Sprint	N/A	Strength
Easy	5→3 min	—	—	Easy	LSD	
Long sprint	45–90 s†	↑	↑	Long sprint	N/A	
Easy	6→3 min	—	—	Easy	LSD	
Repeat VR	20/20/20 s†	↑	↑	Sprint	N/A	Sprint, recover, sprint again
Easy	6→3 min	—	—	Easy	LSD	
Repeat KK	10/10 s†	↑	↑	K & K	N/A	'Kick' and 'kick' again
Warm down	5–10 min	—	—	Easy	LSD	

** Over a period of time drop or increase the workout or recovery time so 1→3 means increase from 1 to 3 min over a period of weeks and 3→1 means decrease in the same way. Always start with the recovery at the longest duration and the effort at the shortest duration.

Place training heart rates from pages 42–43 in here.

* Remove these parts of your programme for a shorter/easier workout.

† Having completed the effort, pedal gently for the rest of the minute and begin the next part of the workout at the start of the next minute.

CODES	GEAR/RES	CADENCE
—	Usual/comfortable	Usual/comfortable
↑	A little harder (↑1–2 cogs)	A little higher (↑5 rpm)
↑↑	Moderately harder (↑2–3 cogs)	Moderately higher (↑10 rpm)
↑↑↑	Much harder (↑4–5 cogs)	Much higher (↑15+ rpm)
↓↓↓	Much easier (↓4–6 cogs)	Much lower (↓30 rpm)
↓↓	Moderately easier (↓2–4 cogs)	Moderately lower (↓20 rpm)
↓	A little easier (↓1–2 cogs)	A little lower (↓10 rpm)

7

SPIN WORKOUT: Sub ⑦   **AIM:** Sprint (anaerobic) speed   **TOTAL TIME:** 83 min
       (1,5,6,7,9)   *47 min

EXTRA INFORMATION

TRAIN TYPE	DURATION	GEAR	CADENCE	EFFORT	HEART RATE	COMMENTS
Warm up	5–10 min	—	—	Easy	LSD	
Overspeed*	10 s†	↓↓↓	↑↑↑	Leg speed	N/A	
Easy*	2 min	—	—	Easy	LSD	
Overspeed	10 s†	↓↓↓	↑↑↑	Leg speed	N/A	
Easy	5 min	—	—	Easy	LSD	
Up tempo	3 min	—	—	Tempo	UT	
Flat sprint	20–30 s†	↑	↑	Sprint (IS)	N/A	Top speed
Easy	5 min	—	—	Easy	LSD	
Up tempo*	3 min	—	—	Tempo	UT	
Repeat VR*	20/20/20 s†	—	—	Sprint	N/A	Sprint, recover, sprint again
Easy*	5 min	—	—	Easy	LSD	
AT	3 min	—	—	Hard	AT	
Flat sprint	20–30 s†	↑	↑	Sprint (IS)	N/A	
Easy*	5 min	—	—	Easy	LSD	
AT*	3 min	—	—	Hard	AT	
Repeat KK*	10/10 s†	—	—	K & K	N/A	'Kick' and 'kick' again
Easy	5 min	—	—	Easy	LSD	
Up tempo	4 min	—	—	Tempo	UT	
Flat sprint*	20–30 s†	↑ then —	↑	Sprint (IS)	N/A	Strength
Easy	5 min	—	—	Easy	LSD	
AT	4 min	—	—	Hard	AT	
Sprint (ES)*	45–90 s†	—	—	Long sprint	N/A	Long sprint
Easy*	1 min	—	—	Easy	LSD	
Repeat KK*	10/10 s†	—	—	K & K	N/A	'Kick' and 'kick' again
Warm down	5–10 min	—	—	Easy	LSD	

*** Remove these parts of your programme
for a shorter/easier workout.**

CODES	GEAR/RES	CADENCE
—	Usual/comfortable	Usual/comfortable
↑	A little harder (↑1–2 cogs)	A little higher (↑5 rpm)
↑↑	Moderately harder (↑2–3 cogs)	Moderately higher (↑10 rpm)
↑↑↑	Much harder (↑4–5 cogs)	Much higher (↑15+ rpm)
↓↓↓	Much easier (↓4–6 cogs)	Much lower (↓30 rpm)
↓↓	Moderately easier (↓2–4 cogs)	Moderately lower (↓20 rpm)
↓	A little easier (↓1–2 cogs)	A little lower (↓10 rpm)

Place training heart rates
from pages 42–43 in here.

**† Having completed the
effort, pedal gently for
the rest of the minute
and begin the next part
of the workout at the
start of the next minute.**

7

SPIN WORKOUT: Sub ⑦ (1,7)

AIM: Sprint (anaerobic) speed

TOTAL TIME: 25–89 min

TRAIN TYPE	SET	REP	DURATION	REST**	GEAR	CADENCE	GRAD/RES	HEART RATE	COMMENTS
Warm up	1–6x	1x	20 s	—	42 x 18–21	75–85	0% or 1	LSD	Easy
		1x	20 s	—	42 x 18–21	85–95	0% or 1	LSD	Easy
		1x	10 s	—	42 x 18–21	95–105	0% or 1	LSD	Easy
		1x	10 s	—	42 x 18–21	105–125	0% or 1	LSD	Easy
Flat sprint	—	1–3x	20–30 s†	2 min	52 x 14–18	85→130	0% or 1	N/A	Sprint top speed (IS)
Easy	—	1x	5–10 min	—	42 x 16–18	85–95	0% or 1	LSD	Easy
Uphill sprint	—	1–2x	20–30 s†	2 min	42 x 14–16	85→105	3–5% or 2–4	N/A	Sprint strength (IS)
Easy*	—	1x	5–10 min	—	42 x 16–18	85–95	0% or 1	LSD	Easy
Crest sprint	—	1–2x	20–30 s†	2 min	42 x 14–16	85→125	3% or 2→0% or 1	N/A	Sprint strength (IS)
Easy*	—	1x	5–10 min	—	42 x 16–18	85–95	0% or 1	LSD	Easy
Flat sprint	—	1–2x	20–30 s†	2 min	52 x 14–18	85→130	0% or 1	N/A	Sprint top speed (IS)
Easy	—	1x	5–10 min	—	42 x 16–18	85–95	0% or 1	LSD	Easy
Sprint	—	1–2x	30–60 s†	2 min	52 x 15–18	85→120	0% or 1	N/A	Long sprint, extensive (ES)
Warm down	—	1x	5–10 min	—	42 x 18–21	85–95	0% or 1	LSD	Easy

EXTRA INFORMATION

Place training heart rates from pages 42–43 in here.

* Remove these parts of your programme for a shorter/easier workout.

** Rest means easy active recovery pedalling (42 x 18–21).

† Having completed the effort, pedal gently for the rest of the minute and begin the next part of the workout at the start of the next minute.

SPIN WORKOUT: Sub ⑦ (1,7)

AIM: Sprint (anaerobic) speed

TOTAL TIME: 36–84 min

TRAIN TYPE	SET	REP	DURATION	REST**
Warm up	—	1x	5 min	—
Sprint	—	1–2x	20–30 s†	2 min
Easy	—	1x	5–10 min	—
Sprint	—	1–2x	30–60 s†	3 min
Easy	—	1x	5–10 min	—
Repeat	1x	1x	10–20 s	10–20 s
		1x	10–20 s†	2 min
Easy	—	1x	5–10 min	—
Repeat VR*	1x	1x	10–20 s	20–30 s
		1x	10–20 s	10–20 s
		1x	20–30 s†	2 min
Easy*	—	1x	5–10 min	—
Repeat KK*	1x	1x	10–20 s	—
		1x	10–20 s†	5 min
Warm down	—	1x	5–10 min	—

EXTRA INFORMATION

GEAR	CADENCE	GRAD/RES	HEART RATE	COMMENTS
42 x 18–21	85–95	0% or 1	LSD	Easy
52 x 14–18	85→120	0% or 1	N/A	Sprint top speed (IS)
42 x 16–18	85–95	0% or 1	LSD	Easy
52 x 14–18	85→120	3% or 2	N/A	Sprint top speed (IS)
42 x 16–18	85–95	0% or 1	LSD	Easy
52 x 14–18	85→120	0% or 1	N/A	Sprint, recover, sprint again
52 x 14–18	85→120	0% or 1	N/A	
42 x 16–18	85–95	0% or 1	LSD	Easy
52 x 14–18	85→120	0% or 1	N/A	Sprint, recover, sprint, recover,
52 x 14–18	85→120	3% or 2	N/A	sprint again
52 x 14–18	85→120	0% or 1	N/A	
42 x 16–18	85–95	0% or 1	LSD	Easy
52 x 14–18	85→120	0% or 1	N/A	'Kick' and 'kick' again
52 x 14–18	85→120	3% or 2	N/A	
42 x 18–21	85–95	0% or 1	LSD	Easy

Place training heart rates from pages 42–43 in here.

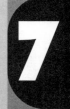

* **Remove these parts of your programme for a shorter/easier workout.**

** **Rest means easy active recovery pedalling (42 x 18–21).**

† **Having completed the effort, pedal gently for the rest of the minute and begin the next part of the workout at the start of the next minute.**

8. Power training — explosive acceleration

Power training improves your explosive ability (acceleration and sprinting). This subphase can occur once or twice a week over a 1–4-week period. The subphase is emphasised towards the end of Speed training.

SPECIFICS: Explosive acceleration. Accelerations ('jumps' and 'kicks') at a normal pace in a normal gear.

EFFORT: *During:* Can't think to converse (100 percent effort); high muscular effort.

Between: Easy conversation pace (50–60 percent effort); easy muscular effort.

BIKE: Explosive accelerations as you would use when attacking at lower speeds or 'jumping', and accelerations where you explosively attack at high speeds or 'kicking'. There are three variations:

Accelerations: Big gear windouts from a freewheeling rolling speed (5–20 kph) and accelerating up till you are on top of the gear (there is no more heavy to medium muscular effort to turn the gear over); 20–100 m;

Power climbs: Come down a hill in a big gear at high cadence (wound out) into a dip and with the momentum accelerate up the other side of a short hill (no more than 100–200 m) until you start to labour the gear, then pull out. Don't get bogged down or buried by the gear; pull out before this happens;

Kick and kick: 'Kick' or 'jump' for the line and while at top speed 'kick' again with 50 m to go.

Duration: 20–200-m reps.

During: Explosive efforts — reps.

Gears: Big gears; 52 or 53 x 12–18.

Cadence: 0 (not pedalling)

Acceleration: Freewheeling → approx. 160 rpm;

Power climb: 95 →105 rpm;

Kick and kick: 95 →140 rpm.

Between: Easy riding.

Gears: Easy/small gears — small chainring; 39 or 42 x 16–21.

Cadence: 85–95 rpm for time trialling, triathlon and duathlon; 95–105 rpm for road cycling and triathlon with legal drafting.

Training heart rate = During: N/A   Between:

(LSD: 60–75 percent HR^{max}).

See pages 42–43 for reference table.

NOTE: Power sprints are performed at a higher resistance (bigger gear, higher gradient) than extensive and intensive sprints (watch for wheel slippage on the trainer).

SPIN WORKOUT: Sub ⑧
(1,8,9)

AIM: Power and explosive acceleration training

TOTAL TIME: 38 min

EXTRA INFORMATION

TRAIN TYPE	DURATION*	GEAR/RES	CADENCE	EFFORT	HEART RATE	COMMENTS
Warm up	10 min	—	—	Easy	LSD	
Power sprints	10 s†	↑	↑	Explosive rolling	N/A	Rolling = higher
Easy	2 min	—	—	Easy	LSD	speeds (20–50 kph)
Power sprints	10 s†	↑	↑	Explosive rolling	N/A	
Easy	2 min	—	—	Easy	LSD	
Overspeed	10 s†	↓↓↓	↑↑↑	Leg speed	N/A	Standing = lower
Power sprints	10 s†	↑↑	↑↑	Explosive rolling	N/A	speeds (5–10 kph)
Easy	2 min	—	—	Easy	LSD	
Power acceleration	10 s†	↑↑	↑↑	Explosive standing	N/A	
Easy	2 min	—	—	Easy	LSD	
Power acceleration	10 s†	↑↑↑	↑↑	Explosive standing	N/A	
Easy	2 min	—	—	Easy	LSD	
Power acceleration	10 s†	↑↑	↑↑	Explosive standing	N/A	
Power sprints	10 s†	↑	↑↑	Explosive rolling	N/A	
Warm down	10 min	—	—	Easy	LSD	

† **Having completed the effort, pedal gently for the rest of the minute and begin the next part of the workout at the start of the next minute.**

Place training heart rates from pages 42–43 in here.

CODES	GEAR/RES	CADENCE
—	Usual/comfortable	Usual/comfortable
↑	A little harder (↑1–2 cogs)	A little higher (↑5 rpm)
↑↑	Moderately harder (↑2–3 cogs)	Moderately higher (↑10 rpm)
↑↑↑	Much harder (↑4–5 cogs)	Much higher (↑15+ rpm)
↓↓↓	Much easier (↓4–6 cogs)	Much lower (↓30 rpm)
↓↓	Moderately easier (↓2–4 cogs)	Moderately lower (↓20 rpm)
↓	A little easier (↓1–2 cogs)	A little lower (↓10 rpm)

8

SPIN WORKOUT: Sub ⑧
(1,7,8,9)

AIM: Power and explosive acceleration training

TOTAL TIME: 66 min
*38 min

EXTRA INFORMATION

TRAIN TYPE	DURATION*	GEAR/RES	CADENCE	EFFORT	HEART RATE	COMMENTS
Warm up	5–10 min	—	—	Easy	LSD	
Overspeed	10 s†	↓↓↓	↑↑↑	Leg speed	N/A	see pg 134
Easy	2 min	—	—	Easy	LSD	
Overspeed*	10 s†	↓↓↓	↑↑↑	Leg speed	N/A	
Easy*	2 min	—	—	Easy	LSD	
Power sprints	10 s†	↑	↑	Explosive rolling	N/A	*** Remove these parts of your programme for a shorter/easier workout.**
Easy	2 min	—	—	Easy	LSD	
Power sprints*	10 s†	↑	↑	Explosive rolling	N/A	
Easy*	2 min	—	—	Easy	LSD	
Power acceleration*	10 s†	↑↑	↑	Explosive standing	N/A	
Easy*	2 min	—	—	Easy	LSD	**† Having completed the effort, pedal gently for the rest of the minute and begin the next part of the workout at the start of the next minute.**
Power acceleration	10 s†	↑↑	↑	Explosive standing	N/A	
Easy	2 min	—	—	Easy	LSD	
Repeat KK	10 s/10 s†	↑↑	↑	Explosive speed	N/A	
Easy	4 min	—	—	Easy	LSD	
Flat sprint (IS)*	20–30 s†	—	—	Sprint top speed	N/A	
Easy*	4 min	—	—	Easy	LSD	
Flat Sprint (IS)	20–30 s†	↑	↑	Sprint top speed	N/A	
Easy	4 min	—	—	Easy	LSD	
Long sprint (ES)	45–90 s†	↑	↑	Long sprint	N/A	
Easy	4 min	—	—	Easy	LSD	
Power acceleration	10 s†	↑↑	↑	Explosive standing	N/A	
Easy	2 min	—	—	Easy	LSD	
Power sprint*	10 s†	↑	↑	Explosive rolling	N/A	
Easy*	2 min	—	—	Easy	LSD	
Overspeed*	10 s†	↓↓↓	↑↑↑	Leg speed	N/A	
Warm down	5–10 min	—	—	Easy	LSD	

Place training heart rates from pages 42–43 in here.

CODES	GEAR/RES	CADENCE
—	Usual/comfortable	Usual/comfortable
↑	A little harder (↑1–2 cogs)	A little higher (↑5 rpm)
↑↑	Moderately harder (↑2–3 cogs)	Moderately higher (↑10 rpm)
↑↑↑	Much harder (↑4–5 cogs)	Much higher (↑15+ rpm)
↓↓↓	Much easier (↓4–6 cogs)	Much lower (↓30 rpm)
↓↓	Moderately easier (↓2–4 cogs)	Moderately lower (↓20 rpm)
↓	A little easier (↓1–2 cogs)	A little lower (↓10 rpm)

8

SPIN WORKOUT: Sub ⑧ (1,8) **AIM:** Power and explosive acceleration training **TOTAL TIME:** 27–83 min

EXTRA INFORMATION

TRAIN TYPE	SET	REP	DURATION	REST**	GEAR	CADENCE	GRAD/RES	HEART RATE	COMMENTS
Warm up	—	1x	5 min	—	42 x 18–21	85–95	0% or 1	LSD	Easy
Power acc	—	1x	10 s†	2 min	52 x 14–18	Stand→140	3% or 2	N/A	Jump — explosive standing
Easy	—	1x	5–10 min	—	42 x 16–18	85–95	0% or 1	LSD	Easy
Power sprint	—	1x	10 s†	2 min	52 x 12–16	85→130	3% or 3	N/A	Explosive rolling — stand
Easy*	—	1x	5–10 min	—	42 x 16–18	85–95	0% or 1	LSD	Easy
Power acc*	—	1x	10 s†	2 min	52 x 14–18	Stand→140	3% or 2	N/A	Seated — explosive seated
Easy*	—	1x	5–10 min	—	42 x 16–18	85–95	0% or 1	LSD	Easy
Power sprint*	—	1x	10 s†	2 min	52 x 12–16	85→130	3% or 2	N/A	Seated — explosive rolling
Easy*	—	1x	5–10 min	—	42 x 16–18	85–95	0% or 1	LSD	Easy
Repeat PA*	1x	{ 1x	10 s	20–30 s	52 x 14–18	Stand→140	3% or 2	N/A	Jump — explosive standing
Power sprint*		{ 1x	10 s	10–20 s	52 x 12–16	85→130	3% or 2	N/A	Kick — explosive rolling
Power sprint**		{ 1x	10 s†	2 min	52 x 12–16	85→130	5% or 4	N/A	Kick — explosive rolling
Easy*	—	1x	5–10 min	—	42 x 16–18	85–95	0% or 1	LSD	Easy
Repeat	1x	{ 1x	10 s	—	52 x 14–18	Stand→140	3% or 2	N/A	Kick/Kick explosive standing
PA/PS		{ 1x	10 s†	5 min	52 x 12–16	85→130	3% or 2	N/A	Explosive rolling
Warm down	—	1x	5 min	—	42 x 18–21	85–95	0% or 1	LSD	Easy

Place training heart rates from pages 42–43 in here.

PA/PS = Power accelerations/Power sprints

* Remove these parts of your programme for a shorter/easier workout.

** Rest means easy active recovery pedalling (42 x 18–21).

† Having completed the effort, pedal gently for the rest of the minute and begin the next part of the workout at the start of the next minute.

SPIN WORKOUT: Sub ⑧ (1,5,6,7,8)

AIM: Power and explosive acceleration training   **TOTAL TIME:** 32–54 min

EXTRA INFORMATION

TRAIN TYPE	SET	REP	DURATION	REST*	GEAR	CADENCE	GRAD/RES	HEART RATE	COMMENTS
Warm up	1–2x	1x	20 s	—	42 x 18–21	75–85	0% or 1	LSD	Easy
		1x	20 s	—	42 x 18–21	85–95	0% or 1	LSD	Easy
		1x	10 s	—	42 x 18–21	95–105	0% or 1	LSD	Easy
		1x	10 s	—	42 x 18–21	105–125	0% or 1	LSD	Easy
	1x	1x	1 min	—	42 x 18–21	85–95	0% or 1	LSD	Easy
		1x	1 min	—	42 x 16–18	85–95	0% or 1	LSD	Easy
		1x	1 min	—	42 x 14–16	85–95	0% or 1	LSD	Easy
	—	1x	1 min	—	42 x 18–21	85–95	0% or 1	LSD	Easy
Power acc	—	1–2x	10 s†	2 min	52 x 14–18	Stand→140	3% or 2	N/A	Explosive standing
Power sprints	—	1x	10 s†	2 min	52 x 12–16	85→130	3% or 2	N/A	Explosive rolling
Sprint	—	1–2x	20–30 s†	2 min	52 x 14–18	85→130	0% or 1	N/A	Sprint top speed (IS)
Sprint	—	1x	30–60 s†	4 min	52 x 15–18	85→120	0% or 1	N/A	Long sprint (ES)
AT	—	1–2x	2 min	4 min	52 x 14–16	85–95	0% or 1	AT	Hard
Up tempo	—	1x	2–6 min	—	42 x 12–16	85–95	0% or 1	UT	Tempo
Warm down	—	1x	5–10 min	—	42 x 18–21	85–95	0% or 1	LSD	Easy

Place training heart rates from pages 42–43 in here.

* **Rest means easy active recovery pedalling (42 x 18–21).**

† **Having completed the effort, pedal gently for the rest of the minute and begin the next part of the workout at the start of the next minute.**

SPIN WORKOUT: Sub ⑧
(1,2,5,6,7,8)

AIM: Power and explosive acceleration training

TOTAL TIME: 40–61 min

TRAIN TYPE	SET	REP	DURATION	REST*
Warm up	—	1x	5 min	—
Power acc	—	1–2x	10 s†	2 min
Power sprint	—	1x	10 s†	2 min
Sprint	—	1–2x	20–30 s†	2 min
Sprint	—	1x	30–60 s†	2 min
AT	—	1–2x	3 min	3 min
Up tempo	—	1x	5 min	3 min
Hills	—	1–2x	2 min	2 min
Warm down	—	1x	5–10 min	—

EXTRA INFORMATION

GEAR	CADENCE	GRAD/RES	HEART RATE	COMMENTS
42 x 18–21	85–95	0% or 1	LSD	Easy
52 x 14–18	Stand→140	3% or 2	N/A	Explosive standing
52 x 12–16	85→130	3% or 2	N/A	Explosive rolling
52 x 14–18	85→130	0% or 1	N/A	Sprint top speed (IS)
52 x 15–18	85→120	0% or 1	N/A	Long sprint (ES)
52 x 14–16	85–95	0% or 1	LSD	Hard
42 x 12–16	85–95	0% or 1	LSD	Tempo
42 x 14–16	40–60	3–5% or 2–4	N/A	Grunt
42 x 18–21	85–95	0% or 1	LSD	Easy

Place training heart rates from pages 42–43 in here.

* **Rest means easy active recovery pedalling (42 x 18-21).**

† **Having completed the effort, pedal gently for the rest of the minute and begin the next part of the workout at the start of the next minute.**

9. Overspeed training — muscle contraction speed improvement

Overspeed training is used to improve muscle contraction speed, thereby further enhancing top speed sprinting ability.

SPECIFICS: Short downhill sprint intervals or motorpacing (drafting behind a motor vehicle) at above race-pace speed to enhance muscle contraction speed. Downhill spinning sprints at high speed in a small gear.

EFFORT: *During:* Easy (50–60 percent); low muscular effort.

 Between: Easy conversation pace (50–60 percent effort); easy muscular effort.

BIKE: Small gear windouts or sustained high-cadence training. There are two variations:

Downhill spinning sprint: Accelerating down a hill in a small gear at a very high cadence (120–220 rpm) and trying to maintain a smooth pedal action by learning to contract and relax the muscles quickly (20–200 m).

Sustained high cadence: Riding for periods of 5–60 minutes at elevated cadences (usually 110–130 rpm).

 Duration: 20–200-m reps.

 During: Downhill spinning sprints and sustained high-cadence. Gears: Small gears; 39 or 42 x 18–21.

 Cadence: Downhill spinning sprints: 120–220 rpm;

 Sustained high cadence: 110–130 rpm.

 Between: Easy riding. Gears: Easy/small gears — small chainring; 39 or 42 x 16–21.

 Cadence: 85–95 rpm for time trialling, triathlon and duathlon; 95–105 rpm for road cycling and triathlon with legal drafting.

Training heart rate = During: N/A   Between:

(LSD: 60–75 percent HR^{max}).

See pages 42–43 for reference table

NOTE: The stationary trainer has to be completely unloaded (either very small gears or very little resistance).

PROGRAMME 9A   INTERMEDIATE SPORT

SPIN WORKOUT: Sub ⑨ **AIM:** Overspeed **TOTAL TIME:** 61 min
(1,7,8,9)   training and   *31 min
sprint maintenance

EXTRA INFORMATION

TRAIN TYPE	DURATION	GEAR	CADENCE	EFFORT	HEART RATE	COMMENTS
Warm up	5–10 min	—	—	Easy	LSD	*** Remove these parts of your programme for a shorter/easier workout.**
Overspeed	10 s†	↓↓↓	↑↑↑	Leg speed	N/A	
Easy	2 min	—	—	Easy	LSD	
Overspeed	10 s†	↓↓↓	↑↑↑	Leg speed	N/A	
Easy	2 min	—	—	Easy	LSD	
Overspeed*	10 s†	↓↓↓	↑↑↑	Leg speed	N/A	**† Having completed the effort, pedal gently for the rest of the minute and begin the next part of the workout at the start of the next minute.**
Easy*	2 min	—	—	Easy	LSD	
Power sprint	10 s†	↑	↑	Explosive rolling	N/A	
Easy	2 min	—	—	Easy	LSD	
Power acceleration	10 s†	↑↑	↑	Explosive standing	N/A	
Easy	2 min	—	—	Easy	LSD	
Intensive sprint	20–30 s†	↑	↑	Top speed	N/A	
Easy	4 min	—	—	Easy	LSD	
Extensive sprint*	45–90 s†	↑	↑	Long sprint	N/A	
Easy*	4 min	—	—	Easy	LSD	
Intensive sprint*	20–30 s†	↑	↑	Top speed	N/A	
Easy*	4 min	—	—	Easy	LSD	
Power acceleration*	10 s†	↑↑	↑	Explosive standing	N/A	
Easy*	2 min	—	—	Easy	LSD	
Power sprint*	10 s†	↑	↑	Explosive rolling	N/A	
Easy*	2 min	—	—	Easy	LSD	
Overspeed	10 s†	↓↓↓	↑↑↑	Leg speed	N/A	
Easy	2 min	—	—	Easy	LSD	
Overspeed	10 s†	↓↓↓	↑↑↑	Leg speed	N/A	
Warm down	5–10 min	—	—	Easy	LSD	

Place training heart rates from pages 42–43 in here.

CODES	GEAR/RES	CADENCE
—	Usual/comfortable	Usual/comfortable
↑	A little harder (↑1–2 cogs)	A little higher (↑5 rpm)
↑↑	Moderately harder (↑2–3 cogs)	Moderately higher (↑10 rpm)
↑↑↑	Much harder (↑4–5 cogs)	Much higher (↑15+ rpm)
↓↓↓	Much easier (↓4–6 cogs)	Much lower (↓30 rpm)
↓↓	Moderately easier (↓2–4 cogs)	Moderately lower (↓20 rpm)
↓	A little easier (↓1–2 cogs)	A little lower (↓10 rpm)

8

SPIN WORKOUT: Sub ⑨ **AIM:** Overspeed **TOTAL TIME:** 32–42 min
(1,9)   training   or 27–60 min

EXTRA INFORMATION

TRAIN TYPE	DURATION*	GEAR	CADENCE	EFFORT	HEART RATE	COMMENTS
Warm up	5–10 min	—	—	Easy	LSD	† **Having completed**
Overspeed	10†	↓↓↓	↑↑↑	Leg speed	N/A	**the effort, pedal**
Easy	2 min	—	—	Easy	LSD	**gently for the rest**
Overspeed	10 s†	↓↓↓	↑↑↑	Leg speed	N/A	**of the minute and**
Easy	2 min	—	—	Easy	LSD	**begin the next part**
Overspeed	10 s†	↓↓↓	↑↑↑	Leg speed	N/A	**of the workout at**
Easy	2 min	—	—	Easy	LSD	**the start of the**
Overspeed	10 s†	↓↓↓	↑↑↑	Leg speed	N/A	**next minute.**
Easy	2 min	—	—	Easy	LSD	
Overspeed	10 s†	↓↓↓	↑↑↑	Leg speed	N/A	
Easy	2 min	—	—	Easy	LSD	
Overspeed	10 s†	↓↓↓	↑↑↑	Leg speed	N/A	
Easy	2 min	—	—	Easy	LSD	
Overspeed	10 s†	↓↓↓	↑↑↑	Leg speed	N/A	
Easy	2 min	—	—	Easy	LSD	
Overspeed	10 s†	↓↓↓	↑↑↑	Leg speed	N/A	
Warm down	5–10 min	—	—	Easy	LSD	
OR						
Warm up	5→10 min	—	—	Easy	LSD	
Overspeed tempo	5→10 min	↓↓↓	↑↑	Leg speed	Tempo	
Easy	5→1 min	—	—	Easy	LSD	
Overspeed tempo	5→10 min	↓↓↓	↑↑	Leg speed	Tempo	
Easy	5→1 min	—	—	Easy	LSD	
Overspeed tempo	5→10 min	↓↓↓	↑↑	Leg speed	Tempo	
Warm down	5→10 min	—	—	Easy	LSD	

Place training heart rates from pages 42–43 in here.

CODES	GEAR/RES	CADENCE
—	Usual/comfortable	Usual/comfortable
↑	A little harder (↑1–2 cogs)	A little higher (↑5 rpm)
↑↑	Moderately harder (↑2–3 cogs)	Moderately higher (↑10 rpm)
↑↑↑	Much harder (↑4–5 cogs)	Much higher (↑15⁺ rpm)
↓↓↓	Much easier (↓4–6 cogs)	Much lower (↓30 rpm)
↓↓	Moderately easier (↓2–4 cogs)	Moderately lower (↓20 rpm)
↓	A little easier (↓1–2 cogs)	A little lower (↓10 rpm)

** **Over a period of time drop or increase the workout or recovery time so 1→3 means increase from 1 to 3 min over a period of weeks and 3→1 means decrease in the same way. Always start with the recovery at the longest duration and the effort at the shortest duration.**

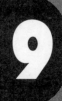

AIM: Overspeed training   **TOTAL TIME:** 41–87 min

SPIN WORKOUT: Sub ⑨ (1,9)

EXTRA INFORMATION

TRAIN TYPE	SET	REP	DURATION	REST**	GEAR	CADENCE	GRAD/RES	HEART RATE	COMMENTS
Warm up	1–6x	1x	20 s	—	42 x 18–21	75–85	0% or 1	LSD	Easy
		1x	20 s	—	42 x 18–21	85–95	0% or 1	LSD	Easy
		1x	10 s	—	42 x 18–21	95–105	0% or 1	LSD	Easy
		1x	10 s	—	42 x 18–21	105–125	0% or 1	LSD	Easy
Overspeed	—	1–4x	10 s†	1 min	42 x 18–21	85→160	0% or 1	N/A	Wind outs; try to remain seated
BG/LG	—	2–4x	1 min	—	52 12–16	40–60	5–7% or 4–6	N/A	See pg 57
			1 min	2 min	42 x 14–18	95→120	0% or 1	N/A	
Overspeed	—	1–2x	10 s†	2 min	42 x 18–21	85→160	0% or 1	N/A	Maximum cadence
Ospd tempo	—	1–4x	1 min	—	42 x 18–21	85–95	0% or 1	N/A	Leg speed tempo
			1 min	—	42 x 18–21	75–105	0% or 1	N/A	
			1 min	—	42 x 18–21	105–115	0% or 1	N/A	
			1 min	—	42 x 18–21	115–125	0% or 1	N/A	
			1 min	—	42 x 18–21	105–115	0% or 1	N/A	
			1 min	—	42 x 18–21	95–105	0% or 1	N/A	
			1 min	—	42 x 18–21	85–95	0% or 1	N/A	
Overspeed	—	1x	10 min	2 min	42 x 18–21	85–95	0% or 1	N/A	If you have sustained the cadence in a previous workout move to the next highest cadence
					42 x 16–18	95–105	0% or 1	N/A	
					42 x 16–18	105–115	0% or 1	N/A	
					42 x 16–18	115–125	0% or 1	N/A	
Overspeed	—	1–2x	10 s†	2 min	42 x 18–21	85→160	0% or 1	N/A	Leg speed
Warm down	—	1x	5 min		42 x 18–21	85–95	0% or 1	LSD	Easy

Place training heart rates from page 42–43 in here.

** Rest means easy active recovery pedalling (42 x 18–21).

† Having completed the effort, pedal gently for the rest of the minute and begin the next part of the workout at the start of the next minute.

SPIN WORKOUT: Sub 9 (1,7,8,9)   **AIM:** Overspeed training and Speed maintenance   **TOTAL TIME:** 22–62 min

EXTRA INFORMATION

TRAIN TYPE	SET	REP	DURATION	REST**	GEAR	CADENCE	GRAD/RES	HEART RATE	COMMENTS
Warm up	1–6x	1x	20 s	—	42 x 18–21	75–85	0% or 1	LSD	Easy
		1x	20 s	—	42 x 18–21	85–95	0% or 1	LSD	Easy
		1x	10 s	—	42 x 18–21	95–105	0% or 1	LSD	Easy
		1x	10 s	—	42 x 18–21	105–125	0% or 1	LSD	Easy
	1–4x	1x	1 min	—	42 x 18–21	85–95	0% or 1	LSD	Easy
		1x	1 min	—	42 x 16–18	85–95	0% or 1	LSD	Easy
		1x	1 min	—	42 x 14–16	85–95	0% or 1	LSD	Easy
		1x	1 min	—	42 x 18–21	85–95	0% or 1	LSD	Easy
Overspeed	—	1–2x	10 s†	2 min	42 x 18–21	85→160	0% or 1	N/A	Leg speed
Power acc	—	1–2x	10 s†	2 min	52 x 14–18	Stand→140	3% or 2	N/A	Explosive standing
Power sprint*	—	1x	10 s†	2 min	52 x 12–16	85→140	3% or 2	N/A	Explosive rolling
Flat sprint	—	1–2x	20–30 s†	2 min	52 x 14–18	85→130	0% or 1	N/A	Sprint top speed (IS)
Crest sprint*	—	1x	20–30 s†	2 min	42 x 14–16	85→120	3% or 2→0% or 1	N/A	Sprint strength (IS)
Uphill sprint*	—	1x	20–30 s†	2 min	42 x 14–16	85→105	3–5% or 2–4	N/A	Sprint strength (IS)
Long sprint	—	1x	30–60 s†	2 min	52 x 15–18	85→120	0% or 1	N/A	Long sprint (ES)
Warm down	—	1x	5–10 min	—	42 x 18–21	85–95	0% or 1	LSD	Easy

> Place training heart rates from page 42–43 in here.

* Remove these parts of your programme for a shorter/easier workout.

** Rest means easy active recovery pedalling (42 x 18–21).

† Having completed the effort, pedal gently for the rest of the minute and begin the next part of the workout at the start of the next minute.

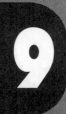

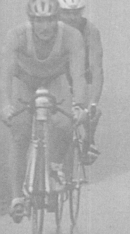

SPIN WORKOUT: Sub ⑨ (1,5,6,7,8,9)   **AIM:** Overspeed training and Speed maintenance   **TOTAL TIME:** 26–58 min

TRAIN TYPE	SET	REP	DURATION	REST*
Warm up	1–6x	1x	20 s	—
		1x	20 s	—
		1x	10 s	—
		1x	10 s	—
Overspeed	—	1–2x	10 s†	1 min
Power sprint	—	1–2x	10 s†	2 min
Flat sprint	—	1–2x	10–20 s†	2 min
Long sprint	—	1x	20–45 s†	2 min
AT	—	1–2x	2 min	2 min
Tempo	—	1x	5 min	—
Warm down	—	1x	5–20 min	—

EXTRA INFORMATION

GEAR	CADENCE	GRAD/RES	HEART RATE	COMMENTS
42 x 18–21	75–85	0% or 1	LSD	
42 x 18–21	85–95	0% or 1	LSD	
42 x 18–21	95–105	0% or 1	LSD	
42 x 18–21	105–125	0% or 1	LSD	
42 x 18–21	85→160	0% or 1	N/A	Little gear windout
52 x 12–16	85→140	3% or 2	N/A	Big gear windout 'jump'
52 x 10–18	85→130	0% or 1	N/A	Top speed sprint (IS)
52 x 15–18	85→120	0% or 1	N/A	Long, extended sprint (ES)
52 x 14–16	85–95	0% or 1	AT	Time trial
42 x 12–16	85–95	0% or 1	UT	Tempo
42 x 18–21	85–95	0% or 1	LSD	Easy

Place training heart rates from pages 42–43 in here.

* Rest means easy active recovery pedalling (42 x 18–21).

† **Having completed the effort, pedal gently for the rest of the minute and begin the next part of the workout at the start of the next minute.**

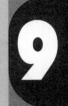

PROGRAMME 10A — INTERMEDIATE AND ADVANCED SPORT

This programme adapts a workout on a stationary cycle trainer to the needs of time-trial training.

SPIN WORKOUT: Sub 6 (1,6)

AIM: High speedwork (time trial)

TOTAL TIME: 46–71 min

EXTRA INFORMATION

TRAIN TYPE	SET	REP	DURATION	REST**	GEAR/RES	CADENCE	EFFORT	HEART RATE	COMMENTS
Warm up	1–2x	1x	1 min	—	—	—	Easy	LSD	
		1x	1 min	—	↑	—	Easy	LSD	
		1x	1 min	—	↑↑	—	Grunt	N/A	
		1x	1 min	—	↑↑↑	—	Grunt	N/A	
	1–2x	1x	20 s	—	—	—	Easy	LSD	
		1x	20 s	—	—	↑	Easy	LSD	
		1x	10 s	—	—	↑↑	Leg speed	N/A	
		1x	10 s	—	—	↑↑↑	Leg speed	N/A	
Easy		1x	5 min	—	—	—	Easy	LSD	
AT		2x	1 min	2 min	—	—	Hard	AT	
Easy		1x	10 min	—	—	—	Easy	LSD	Race pace; focus on rythm
TT		1x	10–20 min	—	—	—	Hard	AT	Time-trial race pace
Warm down		1x	10–20 min	—	—	—	Easy	LSD	

Place training heart rates from pages 42–43 in here.

* **Rest means easy active recovery pedalling (42 x 18–21).**

CODES	GEAR/RES	CADENCE
—	Usual/comfortable	Usual/comfortable
↑	A little harder (↑1–2 cogs)	A little higher (↑5 rpm)
↑↑	Moderately harder (↑2–3 cogs)	Moderately higher (↑10 rpm)
↑↑↑	Much harder (↑4–5 cogs)	Much higher (↑15+ rpm)

EXTRA

SPIN WORKOUT: Sub ⑥   **AIM:** Pursuit and time trial progressive intervals   **TOTAL TIME:** N/A

EXTRA INFORMATION

RACE TYPE	TRAIN TYPE	SET	REP	DURATION	GEAR	CADENCE	EFFORT	HEART RATE	COMMENTS
	Warm up	2x	1x	1 min	—	—	Easy	LSD	
			1x	1 min	←	—	Easy	LSD	
			1x	1 min	↑↑	—	Grunt	N/A	
			1x	1 min	↑↑↑	—	Grunt	N/A	
		3x	1x	20 s	—	—	Easy	LSD	
			1x	20 s	—	↑	Leg speed	N/A	
			1x	10 s	—	↑↑	Leg speed	N/A	
			1x	10 s	—	↑↑↑	Easy	LSD	
	THEN →								
3000 m	Pursuit		10x	200 m	—	—	Race pace	N/A	Rest period 5 min
			6x	500 m	—	—	Race pace	N/A	4 min
			4x	700 m	—	—	Race pace	N/A	3 min
			3x	1000 m	—	—	Race pace	N/A	2 min
			2x	1500 m	—	—	Race pace	N/A	1 min
	OR →								
4000 m	Pursuit		15x	200 m	—	—	Race pace	N/A	Rest period 5 min
			8x	500 m	—	—	Race pace	N/A	4 min
			5x	700 m	—	—	Race pace	N/A	3 min
			4x	1000 m	—	—	Race pace	N/A	2 min
			2x	2000 m	—	—	Race pace	N/A	1 min

Place training heart rates from page 42–43 in here.

(CONTINUED)

EXTRA

This programme adapts a workout on a stationary cycle trainer to the needs of pursuit and time trial progressive intervals.

RACE TYPE	TRAIN TYPE	SET	REP	DURATION	GEAR	CADENCE	EFFORT	HEART RATE	COMMENTS
40 km	TT	OR →	10x	2 km	—	—	Race pace	AT	Rest period: 5 min
			4x	5 km	—	—	Race pace	AT	5 min
			2x	10 km	—	—	Race pace	AT	5 min
			1x	20 km	—	—	Race pace	AT	N/A
20 km	TT	OR →	8x	2 km	—	—	Race pace	AT	Rest period: 5 min
			4x	4 km	—	—	Race pace	AT	4 min
			2x	8 km	—	—	Race pace	AT	2 min
			1x	16 km	—	—	Race pace	AT	N/A
	Warm down		1x	10 min	—	—	Easy	LSD	

Place training heart rates from pages 42–43 in here.

CODES	GEAR/RES	CADENCE
—	Usual/comfortable	Usual/comfortable
↑	A little harder (↑1–2 cogs)	A little higher (↑5 rpm)
↑↑	Moderately harder (↑2–3 cogs)	Moderately higher (↑10 rpm)
↑↑↑	Much harder (↑4–5 cogs)	Much higher (↑15+ rpm)

NOTE: Suggested workout order and progression (e.g. 10 x 2 km, 4 x 5 km, 2 x 10 km, 1 x 20 km) for time trial training are workouts conducted once every 2 weeks (preferred) to once a week over a 4–10 week period.

EXTRA

PROGRAMME 10c

INTERMEDIATE AND ADVANCED SPORT

This programme adapts a workout on a stationary cycle trainer to the needs of a criterium bike race simulation.

AIM: Criterium bike race simulation **TOTAL TIME:** 60 min

SPIN WORKOUT: Sub (6) (1,5,6,7,8)

EXTRA INFORMATION

TRAIN TYPE	SET	REP	DURATION	GEAR/RES	CADENCE	EFFORT	HEART RATE	COMMENTS
Warm up	2x	1x	1 min	—	—	Easy	LSD	
		1x	1 min	←	—	Easy	LSD	
		1x	1 min	⇑⇑	—	Grunt	N/A	
		1x	1 min	⇑⇑⇑	—	Grunt	N/A	
	3x	1x	20 s	—	—	Easy	LSD	
		1x	20 s	—	←	Easy	LSD	
		1x	10 s	—	⇑⇑	Leg speed	N/A	
		1x	10 s	—	⇑⇑⇑	Leg speed	N/A	
Easy		1x	5 min	—	—	Easy	LSD	
Tempo		1x	3 min	—	—	Tempo	UT	
Flat sprint		1x	20 s	←	←	Sprint	N/A	Top speed (IS)
AT		1x	3 min	—	—	Hard	AT	
Long sprint		1x	40 s	—	—	Long sprint	N/A	Sprint (ES)
Tempo		1x	4 min	⇑⇑⇑	—	Tempo/hill	UT	
Power acc	2x	1x	10 s	⇑⇑	—	Kick and	N/A	
Power sprint		1x	10 s†	←	—	kick again	N/A	
AT		1x	3 min	—	—	Hard	AT	
Power acc		1x	10 s†	⇑⇑	—	Kick	N/A	
Flat sprint		1x	20 s	—	—	Sprint	N/A	Sprint (IS)
Warm down		1x	15 min	—	—	Easy	LSD	

Place training heart rates from pages 42–43 in here.

CODES	GEAR/RES	CADENCE
—	Usual/comfortable	Usual/comfortable
←	A little harder (⇑1–2 cogs)	A little higher (⇑5 rpm)
⇑⇑	Moderately harder (⇑2–3 cogs)	Moderately higher (⇑10 rpm)
⇑⇑⇑	Much harder (⇑4–5 cogs)	Much higher (⇑15+ rpm)

† Having completed the effort, pedal gently for the rest of the minute and begin the next part of the workout at the start of the next minute.

EXTRA

'BRICK' TRAINING

PROGRAMME 10D

INTERMEDIATE AND ADVANCED SPORT

This programme adapts a workout on a stationary cycle trainer to the needs of 'brick' training for multisport, triathlon and duathlon.

SPIN WORKOUT: Sub ⑥ **AIM:** Bricks for multisport, triathlon and duathlon **TOTAL TIME:** 25–57 min

EXTRA INFORMATION

TRAIN TYPE	SET	REP	DURATION	GEAR/RES	CADENCE	EFFORT	HEART RATE	COMMENTS
Warm up		1x	5 min	—	—	Easy	LSD	
Bike		1x	5 min	—	—	Easy	LSD	
Transition			—	Fast transition		Fast	N/A	
Run		1x	5 min	N/A	N/A	Easy	LSD	
THEN								
Easy		1x	5 min	—	—	Easy	LSD	
Swim simulation:								
Lat pull over		1x	1 min	N/A	N/A	Hard	N/A	See drawing or use bungy cords
Transition	1–2x	1x	—	Fast transition	—	Fast	N/A	
Bike		1x	2–6 min	—	—	Hard	AT	Add 10 beats to heart rate
Transition			—	Fast transition	N/A	Fast	N/A	
Run		1x	2–4 min	N/A	N/A	Hard	AT	
Warm down		1x	5–10 min	—	—	Easy	LSD	

Place training heart rates from pages 42–43 in here.

TRANSITION PRACTICE

PROGRAMME 10E

INTERMEDIATE AND ADVANCED SPORT

This programme adapts a workout on a stationary cycle trainer to the needs of transition practice for triathlon.

SPIN WORKOUT: Sub ⑥

AIM: Transition practice for triathlon

TOTAL TIME: 18–48 min

EXTRA INFORMATION

TRAIN TYPE	SET	REP	DURATION	GEAR/RES	CADENCE	EFFORT	HEART RATE	COMMENTS
Warm up	—	1x	5 min	—	—	Easy	LSD	
Shower		1x	1 min	N/A	N/A	Shower	N/A	Stand in shower in wetsuit
Transition	1–3x	{	—	Fast transition	Fast transition	Fast	N/A	
Bike		1x	1–5 min	—	—	Easy	LSD	
Transition		}	—	Fast transition	Fast transition	Fast	N/A	
Run		1x	1–5 min	N/A	N/A	Easy	LSD	
Warm down	—	1x	10 min	—	—	Easy	LSD	

Place training heart rates from pages 42–43 in here.

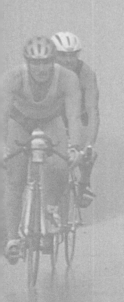

EXTRA

PROGRAMME 10F — INTERMEDIATE AND ADVANCED SPORT

This programme adapts a workout on a stationary cycle trainer to the needs of mountainbike simulation.

AIM: Mountainbike simulation   **TOTAL TIME:** 31–76 min

SPIN WORKOUT: Sub ⑥ (1,2,3,4,6)

EXTRA INFORMATION

TRAIN TYPE	SET	REP	DURATION	GEAR/RES	CADENCE	EFFORT	HEART RATE	COMMENTS
Warm up	—	1x	5 min	—	—	Easy	LSD	
AT		1x	1 min	—	—	Hard	AT	
Off to push		1x	10 s†	Get off and on your bike fast		Jog on spot	N/A	Jog on spot
AT	1–4x	1x	1 min	—	—	Hard	AT	
Off to push		1x	1 min	Get off and on your bike fast		Jog on spot	AT	Jog on spot
Easy	—	1x	5 min	—	—	Easy	LSD	
Hills	—	1x	2 min	⇈	⇊	Grunt	N/A	
Easy	—	1x	2 min	—	—	Easy	LSD	
Hills BG	—	1x	3 min	⇈⇈⇈	⇊⇊⇊	Grunt	N/A	
Easy*	—	1x	2 min	—	—	Easy	LSD	
Hills*	—	1x	4 min	⇈⇈⇈	⇊⇊⇊	Grunt	N/A	
Hills BG*	—	1x	2 min	⇈	⇊	Grunt	N/A	
Flat BG	—	1x	5–10 min	—	—	Grunt	N/A	
Warm down		1x	5–10 min	—	—	Easy	LSD	

(The "Off to push" 10 s† and second AT/Off to push rows are bracketed together as 1–4x)

Place training heart rates from pages 42–43 in here.

CODES	GEAR/RES	CADENCE
—	Usual/comfortable	Usual/comfortable
⇈	Moderately harder (↑2–3 cogs)	Moderately higher (↑10 rpm)
⇈⇈⇈	Much harder (↑4–5 cogs)	Much higher (↑15* rpm)
⇊⇊⇊	Much easier (↓4–6 cogs)	Much lower (↓30 rpm)
⇊	Moderately easier (↓2–4 cogs)	Moderately lower (↓20 rpm)

* Remove these parts of your programme for a shorter/easier workout.

† Having completed the effort, pedal gently for the rest of the minute and begin the next part of the workout at the start of the next minute.

Training for health and fitness

Training to achieve your goals

Fitness can be divided into the following categories:

- aerobic fitness.
- fat loss (see below for body composition assessment).
- health/stress control.
- tone.
- strength.

Let's look at what you need to do to achieve each of these.

Fitness/aerobic endurance

Exercise initially at 60–70 percent of your maximum heart rate (aerobic/fat loss zone) for 4–8 weeks, depending on your level of fitness at the beginning. After that use aspects of 70–80 percent HR^{max} training (high aerobic zone), for another 4–6 weeks, but doing no more than 20 percent of your training at this intensity. Finally do 80–90 percent HR^{max} training (anaerobic threshold zone) for no more than 5–10 percent of your training for 4 weeks.

Overall you should train 3–5 times per week for 30–60 minutes at moderate intensity. You should feel as if you are working, but be able to speak relatively easily while exercising; you should not have a red face following your workout.

Subjectively: 70–80 percent effort.

Recommended number of workout sessions: 2–3 per week.

Activity: any that raises your heart rate to a moderate level, for example walking, running, rowing, steppers, aerobics, circuit classes, high-rep low-weight exercises performed quickly; cycling is very good.

Fat loss

Exercise at 60–70 percent of maximum heart rate (easy intensity; aerobic/fat loss zone) 3–4 times per week. Focus on the duration of your workouts and not the intensity. You should be able to speak continuously while you are working out; if you can't you are training too hard.

Subjectively: 60–70 percent effort.

Recommended number of workouts: 3–4 per week.

Activity: any exercise that raises your heart rate to a moderate level will burn fat. Cycling is very good for this, particularly as it is low impact. Although this type of exercise is at a slightly lower intensity than fitness training, it will also improve fitness.

Always combine your training with a nutritional consultation. If you are already doing a lot of exercise with no fat loss, don't try to do even more exercise. This indicates a fault in your nutrition or dietary patterns.

A lot of people exercise to burn off fat; they may even be working out 6 times a week. Even if you lose the fat you want to, the big question is 'now what?' How do you keep the fat off? If you exercised 6 days a week to get it off, you now have to exercise 6 times a week for the rest of your life to keep it off. A far better long term plan is to combine good nutrition with exercise, both at moderate sustainable levels.

Improvements in well-being, reduction in chronic disease risk and stress

Exercise at 50–60 percent of maximum heart rate (recovery zone) for at least 20–30 minutes, a minimum of 3 times per week. For stress reduction do your workouts when you have time to relax and are not pressured by time constraints. For cardiac rehabilitation do your training in conjunction with the recommendations of your cardiac specialist, and base your training heart rate intensities on the ECG test conducted.

Tone

This is muscle-specific — you must work a particular muscle to tone it. This can be through strength training (which can also increase muscle size to some extent) and/or high-repetition training (which will not increase muscle size); high-repetition training can be performed using weights or without. Strength is not the only way to achieve tone! Cycle training will do this for the legs, but you may require additional exercises for your upper body. Heart rate monitors will not help here.

Strength and size

This usually involves using weight training machines or free weights, generally on low reps and high weights. These exercises have no benefits in terms of fitness but will provide good gains in strength and, if required, size. The exercises are very intense and must be specific to the muscle. To build strength and/or size, workouts supplementary to cycling are necessary. Once again, heart rate monitors will not help.

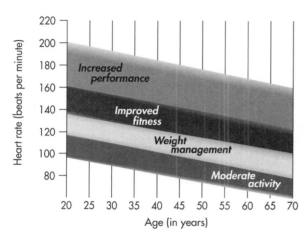

Fig. 9.1: Target range chart

Training intensities

For health and fitness training we can define the following five training zones.

Recovery zone (very easy) — R

The recovery zone is, as its name suggests, a zone where you can actively recover while exercising. The recovery zone is 50–60 percent of maximum heart rate (HR^{max}). The way it helps you recover is by elevating your heart rate slightly at a very easy intensity where there is no stress on the body; the elevated heart rate 'flushes' all the waste products that have been impeding recovery out of the muscles. This intensity is very good for warm-ups and particularly good for warming down, as it helps you to recover from your workout faster.

Aerobic/fat loss zone (easy) — AFL

This zone is the cornerstone of all your training, and where you should spend 80–100 percent of your time. But it's too easy, you say. Maybe it is easy, but that's what you need to make you fit and to help you lose body fat — you don't have to exercise hard. Enjoy the fact that it is easy. It means that you will stick to your programme for far longer, and will find it sustainable throughout your working week. The intensity is 60–70 percent of maximum heart rate, and you should find it very easy to converse.

Don't move into the higher intensities until you have spent between 2 and 12 weeks at this intensity (preferably 6–8 weeks). Your body burns fat better at this intensity so don't waste your time by pushing too hard.

High aerobic zone (moderate tempo) — HA

The high aerobic zone is where an athlete who has been training for 4–8 weeks can train. This is where fitness can be improved significantly.

This training zone occurs at about 70–80 percent of maximum heart rate. You should find it a little difficult to converse, and should feel strong, fast, but in control (as opposed to 'hammering', which is what anaerobic threshold is). This is a tempo intensity: it's faster than cruising, but not enough to hurt. It improves endurance and familiarises the body with a faster pace. Do no more than 5–20 percent of your training at this intensity.

Anaerobic threshold zone (hard) — AT

This zone is as high as someone wanting to exercise for health and fitness should go. It occurs at 80–90 percent of maximum heart rate, and is the fastest you can go for 30 minutes to 1 hour. It should feel difficult to talk.

This intensity should be used only if you have been training for more than 8–12 weeks and want to improve further. Spend no more than 5–10 percent of your workout at this intensity, and do it no more than once or twice a week. It is physically and psychologically very tough and will burn you out if you do too much of it.

A lot of people working without heart rate monitors do their entire workouts at this intensity, thinking that if they train any slower they are barely moving. Wrong! If you spend most of your training time in this zone you will burn out and stop training after 4 to 8 weeks.

Anaerobic threshold training increases your top end endurance ability and aerobic speed. Warm up well before doing this sort of training.

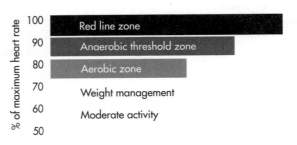

Fig. 9.2: The target training heart rate zones

Red line zone (maximal) — RLZ

The red line zone is the highest intensity, at 90–100 percent of maximum heart rate. This training zone is not necessary for health and fitness training. Red line training is very hard and it is difficult to converse at this intensity. It's the sprinting zone. It should only be used if you are an athlete training for sports that involve sprinting or periods of time in oxygen debt.

The reason it's called the red line zone is that most health and fitness exercisers training at this level are 'red lining' — they are overdoing it and surpassing what is required for their 'motor' (i.e. their body) to operate

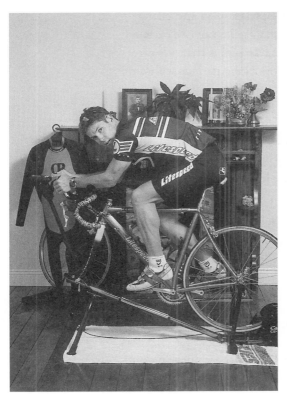

Whether exercising for fitness or fat loss, you should be able to converse easily throughout your whole workout.

properly. Older or sedentary people, and those with heart complaints, should steer clear of this training zone. Repercussions can range from being out of breath to feeling nauseous and dizzy to having a heart attack

Understand what you are doing

Be aware of the purpose of your workouts, their objectives and goals. You should also know what the purpose of each exercise is — why bother putting all that effort and time into your training if you don't know whether it is achieving the results you want?

Calculating your training heart rates

To work out the appropriate heart rates for your own training, see chapter 4, Method 1 (pages 31–33).

Your training programme

You can't train at high levels all year round. You need times of training and times of rest even if you just want to be fit. Therefore you should build your training volumes up then bring them down during a recovery period. Training should build for between 8 and 16 weeks, with a period of 4–6 weeks' recovery from the build-up during which you train lightly. The aerobic/fat loss training should be brought in for 2–8 weeks, followed by 4–6 weeks of high aerobic training, then 4 weeks that includes anaerobic threshold training before going into a recovery period. You've got to crawl before you walk before you run.

A programme change occurs immediately after the recovery period (an easy week). You will progress through the five phases of the programme from recovery zone and aerobic/fat loss zone, making you stronger and more toned on your bike, to high aerobic zone training to anaerobic threshold training. There are two reasons for the progression and change in training — the first is that you will only get so many gains out of a certain type of training, then you need a new type, and the second is that it is rare that an exerciser can sustain continuous training over long periods without requiring some form of recovery.

Choosing your training level

The workouts on the following pages include two different training levels over five different phases of training (providing specific workout quantities). Before you use them you need to select the level that best suits you.

BEGINNER

You are just starting training or just getting back into training. The beginner programmes are those marked 'a' (for example, 5a means phase 5 of your training for a beginner).

EXPERIENCED

You are experienced and have been training for more than 6 months. Programmes for experienced exercisers are marked 'b' (for example, 5b means phase 5 of your training for an experienced exerciser).

Note: Always consult a doctor and have a medical before embarking on a new exercise regime.

Running your programme

WHAT DO I DO? HOW LONG, WHAT TYPE OF TRAINING?

Refer to the following programme (fig 9.3) and look up the number for a particular training day. The number indicates the phase of training you are currently in, phase 1 being easy starting training, through to phase 5 which is 'top end' fitness training. (There is also a phase 6 for people who want to combine cycling with gym or running.) Use the 'a' programmes if you have decided to do a beginner programme, and the 'b' programmes if you are more experienced. Refer to the workouts immediately after the programme for a description of how to do the training and for workouts that you can use (pages 154–65).

HOW HARD DO I GO? HEART RATES

Calculate the correct training heart rates (see Method 1, pages 31–33) and transfer these to the heart rate column in the workouts. You will then have your own individual training intensities for all the varieties of training you will do.

General fitness/Fat loss

Weekly layout:

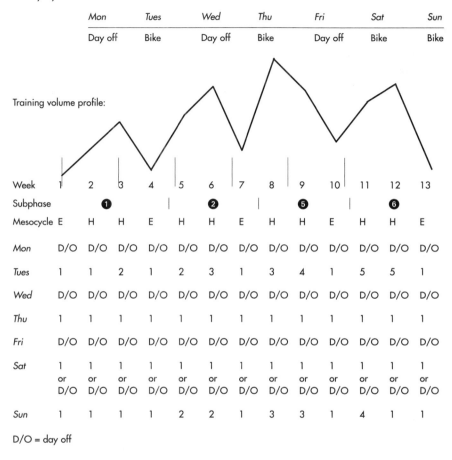

	Mon	Tues	Wed	Thu	Fri	Sat	Sun
	Day off	Bike	Day off	Bike	Day off	Bike	Bike

Training volume profile:

Week	1	2	3	4	5	6	7	8	9	10	11	12	13
Subphase		❶				❷			❺			❻	
Mesocycle	E	H	H	E	H	H	E	H	H	E	H	H	E
Mon	D/O	D/O	D/O	D/O	D/O	D/O	D/O	D/O	D/O	D/O	D/O	D/O	D/O
Tues	1	1	2	1	2	3	1	3	4	1	5	5	1
Wed	D/O	D/O	D/O	D/O	D/O	D/O	D/O	D/O	D/O	D/O	D/O	D/O	D/O
Thu	1	1	1	1	1	1	1	1	1	1	1	1	1
Fri	D/O	D/O	D/O	D/O	D/O	D/O	D/O	D/O	D/O	D/O	D/O	D/O	D/O
Sat	1	1	1	1	1	1	1	1	1	1	1	1	1
	or	or	or	or	or	or	or	or	or	or	or	or	or
	D/O	D/O	D/O	D/O	D/O	D/O	D/O	D/O	D/O	D/O	D/O	D/O	D/O
Sun	1	1	1	1	2	2	1	3	3	1	4	1	1

D/O = day off

Fig. 9.3: Your basic training programme

SPIN WORKOUT: ①a **AIM:** Early Fitness/Fat Loss **TOTAL TIME:** 53 min

EXTRA INFORMATION

DURATION	INTENSITY	HEART RATE	GRAD/RES	COMMENTS
5 min	Easy	AFL	—	Warm up
2 min	V Easy	R	—	Easy pedal — relax
2 min	Easy	AFL	—	Whole pedal stroke
2 min	V Easy	R	—	
4 min	Easy	AFL	—	Push down; see pg 56
2 min	V Easy	R	—	Easy — relax
6 min	Easy	AFL	—	Pull up; see pg 56
2 min	V Easy	R	—	Easy — relax
10 min	Easy	AFL	—	Scrape the mud; see pg 56
2 min	V Easy	R	—	Easy — relax
6 min	Easy	AFL	—	Up and kick the door; see pg 56
2 min	V Easy	R	—	Easy — relax
4 min	Easy	AFL	—	Knees in; see pg 57
2 min	V Easy	R	—	Easy — relax
2 min	Easy	AFL	—	Whole pedal stroke

Place training heart rates from pages 42–43 in here.

See pages 53–58 for comments on technique.

Phase 1: Early fitness and fat loss

PROGRAMME EMPHASIS: The aim of this phase is to begin to get fit and 'burn fat'. You should aim to complete the workout very comfortably in the suggested time. Intensity is not required.

INTENSITY: Easy; aerobic/fat loss and recovery zones.

EFFORT: Easy conversation pace.

SPIN WORKOUT: ①b   **AIM:** Early Fitness/Fat Loss   **TOTAL TIME:** 53 min

EXTRA INFORMATION

DURATION	INTENSITY	HEART RATE	GRAD/RES	COMMENTS
5 min	Easy	AFL	—	Warm up
2 min	V Easy	R	—	Easy pedal — relax
2 min	Easy	AFL	—	Whole pedal stroke
2 min	V Easy	R	—	Easy pedal — relax
2 min	Easy	AFL	—	Fluidity of pedaling
2 min	Tempo	HA	—	Feel strong and fast
2 min	V Easy	R	—	Easy pedal — relax
2 min	Easy	AFL	—	Knees in
2 min	Tempo	HA	—	Feel strong and fast
2 min	Easy	AFL	—	Pull up
2 min	V Easy	R	—	Easy pedal — relax
5 min	Easy	AFL	—	Warm down

Place training heart rates
from pages 42–43 in here.

Phase 1: Early fitness and fat loss

PROGRAMME EMPHASIS: The aim of this phase is to begin to get fit and 'burn
fat'. You should aim to complete the workout very comfortably in the suggested
time. Intensity is not required.
INTENSITY: Easy; aerobic/fat loss and recovery zones.
EFFORT: Easy conversation pace.

2

SPIN WORKOUT: ②a   **AIM:** Building Fitness/Fat Loss Strength Endurance   **TOTAL TIME:** 28 min

EXTRA INFORMATION

DURATION	INTENSITY	HEART RATE	GRAD/RES	COMMENTS
3 min	Easy	AFL	—	Warm up
2 min	V Easy	R	—	Relax — easy pedal
2 min	Grunt	N/A	✓	Slow pedal/high resistance; work your legs
2 min	V Easy	R	—	Relax — easy pedal
2 min	Grunt	N/A	✓✓	Slow pedal/high resistance; work your legs
2 min	V Easy	R	—	Relax — easy pedal
4 min	Grunt	N/A	✓	Slow pedal/high resistance; work your legs
2 min	V Easy	R	—	Relax — easy pedal
4 min	Grunt	N/A	✓✓	Slow pedal/high resistance; work your legs
5 min	V Easy	R	—	Warm down

Place training heart rates from pages 42–43 in here.

Watch your knees and back. Don't overdo the 'grunt' (strength endurance) training. It should be of moderate effort and no more.

Phase 2: Building fitness, fat loss and 'strength'

PROGRAMME EMPHASIS: The aim of this phase is to get fit and 'burn fat', and begin to get stronger on the bike, building tone. You should aim to complete the workout very comfortably in the suggested time. Intensity is not required, but the 'grunt' aspects of the workout will require a moderate degree of muscular effort. ('Grunt' or strength endurance training does not involve a training zone as you are training the muscles not the cardiovascular system.) Phase 1 may also be maintained within this phase.
INTENSITY: Easy; aerobic/fat loss and recovery zones.
EFFORT: Easy conversation pace.

KEY	GRADIENT	RESISTANCE	
—	0	0	Flat
√	2–4%	2	Small Hills
√√	5–7%	3	Med Hills
√√√	8–10%	5	Big Hills

SPIN WORKOUT: ②b   **AIM:** Building Fitness/Fat Loss   **TOTAL TIME:** 45 min
                                Strength Endurance

EXTRA INFORMATION

DURATION	INTENSITY	HEART RATE	GRAD/RES	COMMENTS
5 min	Easy	AFL	—	Warm up
2 min	Grunt	N/A	✓	Slow pedal/high resistance; work your legs
2 min	V Easy	R	—	Relax — easy pedal
2 min	Grunt	N/A	✓	Slow pedal/high resistance; work your legs
2 min	V Easy	R	—	Relax — easy pedal
2 min	Grunt	N/A	✓	Slow pedal/high resistance; work your legs
2 min	MG	N/A	✓✓	More resistance
2 min	V Easy	R	—	Relax — easy pedal
2 min	Grunt		✓	Slow pedal/high resistance; work your legs
2 min	MG	N/A	✓✓	More resistance
2 min	MG	N/A	✓✓✓	More resistance
2 min	V Easy	R	—	Relax — easy pedal
2 min	Grunt	N/A	✓	Slow pedal/high resistance; work your legs
2 min	MG	N/A	✓✓	More resistance
2 min	MG	N/A	✓✓✓	More resistance
2 min	MG	N/A	✓✓✓	More resistance
10 min	V Easy	AFL	—	Warm down

Place training heart rates
from pages 42–43 in here.

MG = More Grunt

KEY	GRADIENT	RESISTANCE	
—	0	0	Flat
✓	2–4%	2	Small Hills
✓✓	5–7%	3	Med Hills
✓✓✓	8–10%	5	Big Hills

Watch your knees and back. Don't overdo the 'grunt' (strength endurance) training. It should be of moderate effort and no more.

Phase 2: Building fitness, fat loss and 'strength'

PROGRAMME EMPHASIS: The aim of this phase is to get fit and 'burn fat', and begin to get stronger on the bike, building tone. You should aim to complete the workout very comfortably in the suggested time. Intensity is not required, but the 'grunt' aspects of the workout will require a moderate degree of muscular effort. ('Grunt' or strength endurance training does not involve a training zone as you are training the muscles not the cardiovascular system.) Phase 1 may also be maintained within this phase.
INTENSITY: Easy; aerobic/fat loss and recovery zones.
EFFORT: Easy conversation pace.

SPIN WORKOUT: ③ a   **AIM:** Strength Endurance and Aerobic Fitness   **TOTAL TIME:** 32 min

EXTRA INFORMATION

DURATION	INTENSITY	HEART RATE	GRAD/RES	COMMENTS
5 min	Easy	AFL	—	Warm up
1 min	Tempo	HA	—	Fast, strong, in control
3 min	V Easy	R	—	Relax — easy pedal
1 min	Tempo	HA	—	Fast, strong, in control
3 min	V Easy	R	—	Relax — easy pedal
1 min	Tempo	HA	—	Fast, strong, in control
3 min	V Easy	R	—	Relax — easy pedal
2 min	Grunt	N/A	✓	Slow pedal/high resistance; work your legs
2 min	V Easy	R	—	Relax — easy pedal
2 min	Grunt	N/A	✓✓	Slow pedal/high resistance; work your legs
2 min	V Easy	R	—	Relax — easy pedal
2 min	Grunt	N/A	✓✓✓	Slow pedal/high resistance; work your legs
5 min	Easy	AFL	—	Warm down

Place training heart rates from pages 42–43 in here.

KEY	GRADIENT	RESISTANCE	
I	0	0	Flat
∨	2-4%	2	Small Hills
∨∨	5-7%	3	Med Hills
∨∨∨	8-10%	5	Big Hills

Phase 3: Strength and tempo fitness

PROGRAMME EMPHASIS: The aim of this phase is to maintain strength on the bike, building tone, and begin to improve fitness at a higher tempo level. You should aim to complete the workout comfortably in the suggested time but you should be going slightly faster than in the previous phases. You should be feeling fast and strong but not struggling, although the 'grunt' aspects of the workout will require a moderate level of muscular effort. ('Grunt' or strength endurance training does not involve a training zone as you are training the muscles not the cardiovascular system.) Previous phases may also be maintained within this phase.
INTENSITY: Tempo; high aerobic zone.
EFFORT: Moderately difficult to converse.

PROGRAMME F

SPIN WORKOUT: ③ b　　**AIM:** Strength Endurance and Aerobic Fitness　　**TOTAL TIME:** 45 min

EXTRA INFORMATION

DURATION	INTENSITY	HEART RATE	GRAD/RES	COMMENTS
5 min	Easy	AFL	—	Warm up
2 min	Tempo	HA	—	Fast, strong, in control
5 min	Easy	AFL	—	Whole pedal stroke
2 min	Tempo	HA	—	Fast, strong, in control
2 min	Easy	AFL	—	Push down
2 min	Grunt	N/A	✓	Slow pedal/high resistance; work your legs
2 min	Easy	AFL	—	Pull up
2 min	Grunt	N/A	✓✓	Slow pedal/high resistance; work your legs
2 min	Easy	AFL	—	Fluidity of pedaling
2 min	Grunt	N/A	✓✓✓	Slow pedal/high resistance; work your legs
2 min	Easy	AFL	—	Knees in
4 min	Grunt	N/A	✓✓	Slow pedal/high resistance; work your legs
4 min	Easy	AFL	—	Whole pedal stroke
2 min	Tempo	HA	—	Fast, strong, in control
2 min	Grunt	N/A	✓	Slow pedal/high resistance; work your legs
5 min	V Easy	AFL	—	Warm down

Place training heart rates from pages 42–43 in here.

KEY	GRADIENT		RESISTANCE	
—	0		0	Flat
✓	2–4%		2	Small Hills
✓✓	5–7%		3	Med Hills
✓✓✓	8–10%		5	Big Hills

Phase 3: Strength and tempo fitness

PROGRAMME EMPHASIS: The aim of this phase is to maintain strength on the bike, building tone, and begin to improve fitness at a higher tempo level. You should aim to complete the workout comfortably in the suggested time but you should be going slightly faster than in the previous phases. You should be feeling fast and strong but not struggling, although the 'grunt' aspects of the workout will require a moderate level of muscular effort. ('Grunt' or strength endurance training does not involve a training zone as you are training the muscles not the cardiovascular system.) Previous phases may also be maintained within this phase.
INTENSITY: Tempo; high aerobic zone.
EFFORT: Moderately difficult to converse.

SPIN WORKOUT: ④a   **AIM:** High Aerobic Fitness   **TOTAL TIME:** 35 min

EXTRA INFORMATION

DURATION	INTENSITY	HEART RATE	GRAD/RES	COMMENTS
5 min	Easy	AFL	—	Warm up
2 min	V Easy	R	—	Easy pedal — relax
1 min	Hard	AT	—	Max 20-min pace at limit of control
3 min	V Easy	R		Easy pedal — relax
1 min	Hard	AT	—	Max 20-min pace at limit of control
3 min	V Easy	R	—	Easy pedal — relax
2 min	Tempo	HA	—	Fast, strong, in control
3 min	V Easy	R	—	Easy pedal — relax
2 min	Tempo	HA	—	Fast, strong, in control
3 min	V Easy	R	—	Easy pedal — relax
10 min	Easy	AFL		Warm down

Place training heart rates
from pages 42–43 in here.

Phase 4: High tempo/aerobic fitness

PROGRAMME EMPHASIS: The aim of this phase is to continue to improve fitness at an even higher tempo level. You should aim to complete the workout comfortably within the suggested time, but you should be going quite hard. You should be feeling fast and strong, and just on the border between going fast and struggling. Previous phases may also be maintained within this phase.

INTENSITY: Hard; anaerobic threshold zone.

EFFORT: Difficult to converse.

PROGRAMME H

SPIN WORKOUT: ④ b **AIM:** Strength Endurance and High Aerobic Fitness **TOTAL TIME:** 37–43 min

EXTRA INFORMATION

DURATION	INTENSITY	HEART RATE	GRAD/RES	COMMENTS
5 min	Easy	AFL	—	Warm up
2 min	Tempo	HA	—	Fast, strong, in control
3→1 min	V Easy	R	—	Easy pedal — relax
2 min	Tempo	HA	—	Fast, strong, in control
3→1 min	V Easy	R	—	Easy pedal — relax
2 min	Hard	AT	—	Max 20-min pace at limit of control
3→1 min	V Easy	R	—	Easy pedal — relax
2 min	Hard	AT	—	Max 20-min pace at limit of control
2 min	Grunt	N/A	✓✓	Slow pedal/high resistance; work your legs
2 min	V Easy	R	—	Easy pedal — relax
2 min	Grunt	N/A	✓✓✓	Slow pedal/high resistance; work your legs
2 min	V Easy	R	—	Easy pedal — relax
2 min	Grunt	N/A	✓✓	Slow pedal/high resistance; work your legs
2 min	Hard	AT	—	Max 20-min pace at limit of control
2 min	V Easy	R	—	Easy pedal — relax
2 min	Tempo	HA	—	Fast, strong, in control
5 min	Easy	R	—	Warm down

Place training heart rates from pages 42–43 in here.

KEY	GRADIENT	RESISTANCE	
—	0	0	Flat
√	2-4%	2	Small Hills
√√	5-7%	3	Med Hills
√√√	8-10%	5	Big Hills

Phase 4: High tempo/aerobic fitness

PROGRAMME EMPHASIS: The aim of this phase is to continue to improve fitness at an even higher tempo level. You should aim to complete the workout comfortably within the suggested time, but you should be going quite hard. You should be feeling fast and strong, and just on the border between going fast and struggling. Previous phases may also be maintained within this phase.

INTENSITY: Hard; anaerobic threshold zone.

EFFORT: Difficult to converse.

PROGRAMME 1   FITNESS/FAT LOSS

SPIN WORKOUT: ⑤ a   **AIM:** High Aerobic Fitness   **TOTAL TIME:** 29 min

EXTRA INFORMATION

DURATION	INTENSITY	HEART RATE	GRAD/RES	COMMENTS
5 min	Easy	AFL	—	Warm up
20 s	Hard	AT	—	Max 20-min pace at limit of control
2 min	Easy	AFL	—	Push down
20 s	Hard	AT	—	Max 20-min pace at limit of control
2 min	V Easy	R	—	Easy pedal — relax
20 s	Hard	AT	—	Max 20-min pace at limit of control
2 min	Easy	AFL	—	Pull up
20 s	Hard	AT	—	Max 20-min pace at limit of control
2 min	V Easy	R	—	Easy pedal — relax
20 s	Hard	AT	—	Max 20-min pace at limit of control
2 min	Easy	AFL	—	Whole pedal stroke
5 min	Hard	AT	—	Max 20-min pace at limit of control
5 min	V Easy	R	—	Warm down

Place training heart rates from pages 42–43 in here.

Phase 5: High aerobic fitness

PROGRAMME EMPHASIS: As in the previous phase, you continue to improve fitness at an even higher tempo level. You should aim to complete the workout comfortably within the suggested time, but you should be going quite hard. You should be feeling fast and strong, and just on the border between going fast and struggling. Previous phases may also be maintained within this phase.

INTENSITY: Hard; anaerobic threshold zone.

EFFORT: Difficult to converse.

SPIN WORKOUT: ⑤ b   **AIM:** High Aerobic Fitness   **TOTAL TIME:** 48–60 min
and Strength Endurance

EXTRA INFORMATION

DURATION	INTENSITY	HEART RATE	GRAD/RES	COMMENTS
10 min	Easy	AFL	—	Warm up
1 min	Hard	AT	—	Max 20-min pace at limit of control
3→1 min	V Easy	R	—	Easy pedal — relax
1 min	Hard	AT	—	Max 20-min pace at limit of control
3→1 min	V Easy	R	—	Easy pedal — relax
1 min	Hard	AT	—	Max 20-min pace at limit of control
3→1 min	V Easy	R	—	Easy pedal — relax
1 min	Hard	AT	—	Max 20-min pace at limit of control
3→1 min	V Easy	R	—	Easy pedal — relax
1 min	Hard	AT	—	Max 20-min pace at limit of control
3→1 min	V Easy	R	—	Easy pedal — relax
2 min	Tempo	HA	—	Fast, strong, in control
2 min	V Easy	R	—	Easy pedal — relax
2 min	Tempo	HA	—	Fast, strong, in control
2 min	V Easy	R	—	Easy pedal — relax
2 min	Grunt	N/A	✓	Slow pedal/high resistance; work your legs
2 min	V Easy	R	—	Easy pedal — relax
2 min	Grunt	N/A	✓✓	Slow pedal/high resistance; work your legs
2 min	V Easy	R	—	Easy pedal — relax
2 min	Grunt	N/A	✓✓✓	Slow pedal/high resistance; work your legs
2 min	V Easy	R	—	Easy pedal — relax
1 min	Hard	AT	—	Max 20-min pace at limit of control
3→1 min	V Easy	R	—	Easy pedal — relax
1 min	Hard	AT	—	Max 20-min pace at limit of control
5 min	Easy	AFL	—	Warm down

KEY

	GRADIENT	RESISTANCE	
—	0	0	Flat
√	2-4%	2	Small Hills
√√	5-7%	3	Med Hills
√√√	8-10%	5	Big Hills

Place training heart rates from pages 42–43 in here.

Phase 5: High aerobic fitness

PROGRAMME EMPHASIS: As in the previous phase, you continue to improve fitness at an even higher tempo level. You should aim to complete the workout comfortably within the suggested time, but you should be going quite hard. You should be feeling fast and strong, and just on the border between going fast and struggling. Previous phases may also be maintained within this phase.

INTENSITY: Hard; anaerobic threshold zone.

EFFORT: Difficult to converse.

PROGRAMME K

SPIN WORKOUT: ⑤ a   **AIM:** High Aerobic Fitness   **TOTAL TIME:** 29 min

EXTRA INFORMATION

DURATION	INTENSITY	HEART RATE	GRAD/RES	COMMENTS
5 min	Easy	AFL	—	Warm up
10 s	Hard	AT	—	Max 20-min pace at limit of control
2 min	Easy	R	—	Easy pedal — relax
1 min	Tempo	HA	—	Fast, strong, in control
2 min	V Easy	R	—	Easy pedal — relax
4 min	Grunt	N/A	✓✓	Slow pedal/high resistance; work your legs
2 min	V Easy	R	—	Easy pedal — relax
2 min	Grunt	N/A	✓✓✓	Slow pedal/high resistance; work your legs
2 min	V Easy	R	—	Easy pedal — relax
1 min	Tempo	HA	—	Fast, strong, in control
2 min	V Easy	R	—	Easy pedal — relax
10 s	Hard	AT	—	Max 20-min pace at limit of control
10 min	Easy	R	—	Warm down

Place training heart rates from pages 42–43 in here.

Run 10–20 min easy or gym **(see programmes on following page).**

Phase 6: Extra cycling with gym/run combination (see page 165).

KEY	GRADIENT	RESISTANCE	
—	0	0	Flat
√	2–4%	2	Small Hills
√√	5–7%	3	Med Hills
√√√	8–10%	5	Big Hills

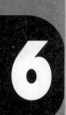

Exercise Programme 1

AIM: Cardiovascular fitness/fat loss and tone
NUMBER OF CIRCUITS: 2–3
PRECAUTION: Be careful if you have back/neck or knee trouble — consult your doctor
HEART RATE: 75–85% HR^{max} for fitness/tone (UT) 60–75% HR^{max} for fat loss/tone (LSD)

EXERCISES	REPS	WEIGHTS (IF APPROPRIATE)
Step ups	15 ea	
Sit ups	20	
Treadmill	1 min	
Bench press	20	
Bike	1 min	
Lat pulldown	20	
Jog on spot	30 ea	
Sit ups	10	
DO AS A FAST CONTINUOUS WORKOUT (MOVE QUICKLY BETWEEN EXERCISES)		

WARM-DOWN: Bike 10 min   Heart rate: 75-50% HR^{max} (LSD)
Stretch

Exercise Programme 2

AIM: Cardiovascular fitness/fat loss
NUMBER OF CIRCUITS: 1
PRECAUTION: Be careful if you have back/neck or knee trouble – consult your doctor
HEART RATE: 75–85% HR^{max} for fitness (UT)
60–75% HR^{max} for fat loss (LSD)

EXERCISES	REPS	WEIGHTS (IF APPROPRIATE)
Stepper	5–15min	
Treadmill (walk or run)	5–15 min	
Rower	5–10	

WARM DOWN: Bike 10 min   Heart rate: 75–50% HR^{max} (LSD)
Stretch
NOTE: If you feel lightheaded or do not feel well during your workout stop immediately and notify your doctor. Do not force yourself to complete the workout. Start slowly and gradually and work towards your targets (circuits, heart rate).
Consult a gym instuctor regarding the exercise and appropriate technique.

Phase 6: Extra cycling with gym/run combination.

Appendix 1

Testing your training

Testing can be conducted to determine what aspects of training you should concentrate on. The main areas that require testing are acceleration and top speed (anaerobic alactic system), sprint speed endurance (anaerobic lactic system), anaerobic threshold and base fitness (aerobic system).

Explosive acceleration and top speed — the highest speed you can achieve — are generally only required by cyclists, although triathlons and multisport events that involve drafting require them to some extent. Sprint speed endurance — your ability to hold a sprint — is required by cyclists, particularly mountain bikers, while anaerobic threshold, maximum steady-state pace (40-km time trial pace), is required by triathletes, duathletes, mountain bikers and cyclists. All the cycling sports require some form of base fitness.

So, we can test:

- Anaerobic alactic 1 system — explosive acceleration: timed sprint (pages 170–73).
- Anaerobic alactic 2 system — top speed: timed sprint (pages 170-73).
- Anaerobic lactic system — sprint speed endurance: timed sprint (pages 170-73).
- Anaerobic threshold: Conconi test (pages 36-40);
- Aerobic system: VO_{2max} test (page 176).
- Strength/strength imbalance testing (pages 51-53).

Tests to do

SYSTEM	TRI	DU	MULTI	MTB	TRI(D)	DU(D)	M(D)	CYCLE
Anaerobic alactic 1								✓
Anaerobic alactic 2				✓	✓	✓	✓	✓
Anaerobic lactic				✓	✓	✓	✓	✓
Anaerobic threshold	✓	✓	✓	✓	✓	✓	✓	✓
Aerobic	✓	✓	✓	✓	✓	✓	✓	✓
Strength imbalances & technique	✓	✓	✓	✓	✓	✓	✓	✓

Key: Tri = triathlon; Du = duathlon; Multi = multisport; MTB = mountainbiking; Tri(D) = triathlon (drafting); Du(D) = duathlon (drafting); M(D) = multisport (drafting); Cycle = cycling.

Test results and analysis

Once your tests are completed, compare them to the table below and graph your results on 'Your assessment table' on page 169.

SYSTEM	EXCELLENT	GOOD	AVERAGE	BELOW AVERAGE	POOR
Anaerobic alactic 1 system – acceleration	M 11 secs F 12 secs	M 12 secs F 13 secs	M 13 secs F 14 secs	M 13 secs F 14 secs	M 14 secs F 15 secs
Anaerobic alactic 2 – top speed	M 18 secs F 19 secs	M 19 secs F 21 secs	M 21 secs F 22 secs	M 22 secs F 23 secs	M 23 secs F 24 secs
Anaerobic lactic – speed endurance	M 32 secs F 37 secs	M 35 secs F 40 secs	M 37 secs F 43 secs	M 38 secs F 44 secs	M 40 secs F 46 secs
Anaerobic threshold – % VO_{2max}	At expected % VO_{2max}	N/A	Less than 5% above or below expected VO_{2max}	5% below expected VO_{2max}	10% above or below expected VO_{2max}
AT — Strength endurance (Points after deflection)	Deflection of 4⁺ points	Deflection of 3–4 points	Deflection of 1–2 points	No Deflection	No Deflection
Aerobic — VO_{2max}	Excellent	Good	Average	Below average	Poor
Strength imbalances	No imbalance	N/A	N/A	Slight imbalance	Very noticeable
Technique	Straight line/ smooth	N/A	N/A	N/A	Wobbly line/ surge

Key: M = Male; F = Female.

Example of performance assessment graph

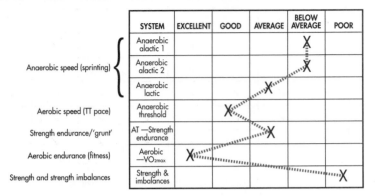

	SYSTEM	EXCELLENT	GOOD	AVERAGE	BELOW AVERAGE	POOR
Anaerobic speed (sprinting)	Anaerobic alactic 1				X	
	Anaerobic alactic 2				X	
	Anaerobic lactic			X		
Aerobic speed (TT pace)	Anaerobic threshold		X			
Strength endurance/'grunt'	AT —Strength endurance			X		
Aerobic endurance (fitness)	Aerobic —VO₂max	X				
Strength and strength imbalances	Strength & imbalances					X

Workouts to do for specific weaknesses

System	Subphases to do	Explanation
Anaerobic alactic 1	8, 9	page 128–39
Anaerobic alactic 2	7 (Intensive sprints)	page 123–27
Anaerobic lactic	7 (Extensive sprints)	page 123–27
Anaerobic threshold	5, 6	page 110–22
Strength endurance	2, 3, 4	page 89–109
Aerobic — VO_{max}	1	page 82–88
Strength imbalances		page 51–53
Technique		page 53–58

Examples of sports assessment graphs

SYSTEM	EXCELLENT	GOOD	AVERAGE	BELOW AVERAGE	POOR
Anaerobic alactic 1	X				
Anaerobic alactic 2	X				
Anaerobic lactic	X				
Anaerobic threshold		X			
AT—Strength endurance		X			
Aerobic —VO₂max		X			
Strength imbalances	X				

Fig A1-1: A good road cyclist (40–80 km multisport bunch riding)

SYSTEM	EXCELLENT	GOOD	AVERAGE	BELOW AVERAGE	POOR
Anaerobic alactic 1					X
Anaerobic alactic 2					X
Anaerobic lactic				X	
Anaerobic threshold	X				
AT—Strength endurance	X				
Aerobic —VO₂max	X				
Strength imbalances	X				

Fig A1-2: A good cyclist, time trialist, triathlete or duathlete (multisport TT)

SYSTEM	EXCELLENT	GOOD	AVERAGE	BELOW AVERAGE	POOR
Anaerobic alactic 1		X			
Anaerobic alactic 2		X			
Anaerobic lactic		X			
Anaerobic threshold		X			
AT—Strength endurance		X			
Aerobic —VO$_{2max}$	X				
Strength imbalances	X				

Fig A1-3: A good tour cyclist

SYSTEM	EXCELLENT	GOOD	AVERAGE	BELOW AVERAGE	POOR
Anaerobic alactic 1					X
Anaerobic alactic 2					X
Anaerobic lactic		X			
Anaerobic threshold	X				
AT—Strength endurance	X				
Aerobic —VO$_{2max}$	X				
Strength imbalances	X				

Fig A1-4: A good mountainbiker

Your assessment table

(as for 'Examples of performance assessment graphs').

SYSTEM	EXCELLENT	GOOD	AVERAGE	BELOW AVERAGE	POOR
Anaerobic alactic 1 – acceleration					
Anaerobic alactic 2 – top speed					
Anaerobic lactic – speed endurance					
Anaerobic threshold (Points after deflection)					
AT — Strength endurance					
Aerobic — VO$_{2max}$					
Strength imbalances					
Technique					

Having completed your table, refer to figs. A1-1 to A1-4 to compare your performance profile with your sport–specific table. This allows you to pinpoint weaknesses. See 'Workouts to do for specific weaknesses', page 168, for a guide to correcting problems.

Appendix 2

Sprint tests — anaerobic alactic and anaerobic lactic system testing

Timed sprint

The timed sprint test involves doing a measured sprint on the road or track over a set distance (500 m). Before doing the sprint, a top speed must be assessed by doing a flying sprint (see below). The 500-m sprint is a sprint from a standing start, where times are taken at 100-m intervals. If time and distance are known, speed can be assessed over acceleration, top speed and speed endurance.

What you need

- Six markers.
- Stopwatch that can take 5 cumulative splits.
- Some measure of distance (industrial tape measure, markings on a velo-drome).
- A timer and assistant to perform the test on the cyclist.

What to do

1. Make sure you have had 1 or 2 days off to recover, so that you perform the test fresh.

2. Measure out and mark 500 m.

3. Measure out and mark each 100 m (i.e. 100 m, 200 m, 300 m, 400 m, 500m). Measure 250 m, then measure 200 m out at right angles and mark it. Make sure the timer always stands at this mark so that they see the cyclist pass each marker from the same angle (see fig A2-1).

4. Warm up for 20 minutes and complete several sprints prior to the test.

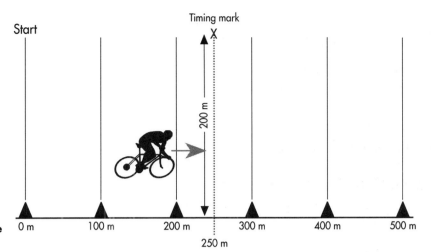

Fig. A2-1: Marking out the sprint course and timing mark

Start

Timing mark
X

200 m

0 m   100 m   200 m   300 m   400 m   500 m

250 m

To assess your top speed, sprint at 100-percent effort through the 200–300-m marks. It is very important to time your sprint correctly to hit top speed between these marks; the mistake generally is to reach top speed too early.

To calculate your top speed use the following equation:

distance (m) / 1000 / time (s) x 60 x 60 = speed (kph)

For example: 100 (m) / 1000 / 6 (s) x 60 x 60 = 60 kph

5. Take 15–20 minutes to recover then perform the standing 500 m.

6. The cyclist needs to be held by an assistant until the timer calls 'go', then the timer times the cyclist as they pass each 100-m marker from the start of the 500-m sprint to the finish (see fig A2-1). The times are then collected and the calculations made. For example:

MARKER	1	2	3	4	5
Distance (m)	111.5	223.0	334.5	446.0	557.5
Time (s)	11.5	19.4	27.4	35.5	44.0
Speed (kph)	36.2	52.5	49.9	48.6	47.4
% top speed	64.3	93.4	88.8	86.5	84.3

To get splits:
Marker 1 = time (s) to get to marker 1   = 11.5
Marker 2 = marker 2 time - marker 1 time = 19.4 - 11.5 = 7.9
Marker 3 = marker 3 time - marker 2 time = 27.4 - 19.4 = 8.0
Marker 4 = marker 4 time - marker 3 time = 35.5 - 27.4 = 8.1
Marker 5 = marker 5 time - marker 4 time = 44.0 - 35.5 = 8.5

Time (2, 3, 4 or 5) - time (1, 2, 3 or 4) = time for 100 metres between (2 and 1, 3 and 2, 4 and 3, 5 and 4).

Speed calculation:

Distance (m) / 1000 / time (s) x 60 x 60 = speed (kph)

Marker 1:
(0–111.5 m) = 111.5 / 1000 / 11.5 x 60 x 60   = 34.9 kph
Marker 2:
(111.5–223 m) = (223 - 111.5) / 1000 / 7.9 x 60 x 60 = 50.8 kph
Marker 3:
(223–334.5 m) = (334.5 - 223) / 1000 / 8.0 x 60 x 60 = 50.2 kph
Marker 4:
(334.5–446 m) = (446 - 334.5) / 1000 / 8.1 x 60 x 60 = 49.6 kph
Marker 5:
(446–557.5 m) = (557.5 - 446) / 1000 / 8.5 x 60 x 60 = 47.2 kph

You can also assess percentage of top speed achieved in each 100 m using the following equation:

Speed in a particular segment / top speed for flying 100 m x 100

   = percentage of top speed achieved

For example, if your top speed is 60 kph, the percentage of top speed achieved in the above example will be:
0–111.5 m = 34.9 / 60 x 100   = 58.2%.
111.5–223.0 m = 50.8 / 60 x 100 = 84.7%.
223.0–334.5 m = 50.2 / 60 x 100 = 83.7%.
334.5–446.0 m = 49.6 / 60 x 100 = 82.7%.
446.0–557.5 m = 47.2 / 60 x 100 = 78.7%.

7. All of this data can then be graphed to illustrate acceleration, top speed and speed endurance.

KEY
Accn = Acceleration (Anaerobic Alactic 1) is time to top speed.
TS = Top speed (Anaerobic Alactic 2) is highest speed achieved.
Speed endurance is how well speed is maintained, or 'drop off' from top speed.

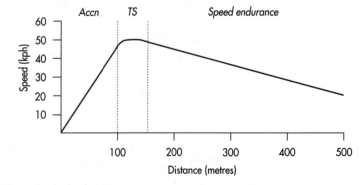

Fig. A2-2: Acceleration (Acc), top speed (TS) and speed endurance

Anaerobic alactic 1 is the time for the 0–100-m interval (i.e. 11.5 seconds in the above example). = ☐ **(Acceleration)**

Anaerobic alactic 2 is the time for the 0–200-m interval (19.4 seconds) = ☐ **(Top speed)**

Anaerobic lactic (no. 3) is the time for the 0–500-m interval (44 seconds) = ☐ **(Speed endurance)**

For analysis, see 'Test Results and analysis', page 167.

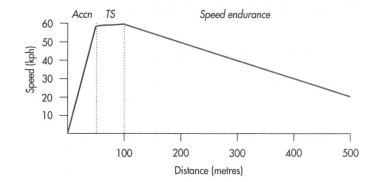

Fig. A2-3: Good acceleration and top speed but speed endurance needs work

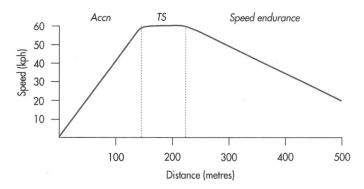

Fig. A2-4: Good top speed but acceleration and speed endurance need work

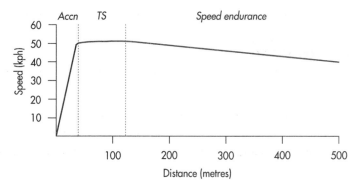

Fig. A2-5: Good acceleration and speed endurance but top speed needs work

Appendix 3

Aerobic system testing

Anaerobic threshold test analysis

If you did an anaerobic threshold test (pages 36–40) to assess training heart rates, you can obtain three other performance measures

1. Strength endurance/muscular endurance.

As you exercise, your body demands fuel, which is oxygen. As the speed/work load is increased your body needs more fuel, so more blood needs to be pumped to carry oxygen to your muscles, increasing your heart rate. The increase is in a straight line in relation to load, until your body can't supply any more oxygen. To keep up the demand at this point, heart rate deflects off the straight line and begins to plateau. To keep going, your body needs to supply some other form of fuel. The only thing that keeps you going is muscular or strength endurance. The longer you last after the deflection and plateau of heart rate, the better your strength endurance.

AT - Strength endurance
(points after deflection)   =   ☐

See 'Test results and analysis' table on page 167 for analysis.

2. Technique

There are two aspects to a poor technical ability in the aerobic threshold test.

a. A fall and rise in the sound of the fan on the stationary trainer: this indicates an uneven distribution of power through the pedal stroke (poor). No change in the sound indicates smooth pedalling (excellent).

b. If you do not change gears correctly during your test on the stationary trainer, your heart rate line in relation to speed/load will be 'wobbly' (poor). A straight line equates to good gear changing (excellent).

3. Percentage of VO_{2max}: are you doing enough speedwork?

You can also assess whether you are doing too much or too little speedwork at different points in your training. This is done by determining anaerobic threshold as a percentage of VO_{2max}. You don't have to know what your VO_{2max} is. In early base AT is low (50-75% of VO_{2max}), whereas near peak AT is much higher (80-90% of VO_{2max}). So depending on where you are in your build-up, you can assess % VO_{2max}. If the percentage is too high for the time of training, you are doing too much speedwork or too much training generally. If the percentage is too low, you aren't doing enough speedwork.

Expected percentages:

Early to Middle Base   =   60-70% of VO_{2max}
Late Base to Early Speed   =   75-80% of VO_{2max}
Middle Speed to Peak   =   80-90% of VO_{2max}

To calculate Percentage of $VO2_{max}$:

$HRAT - HR^{max}$ x 100 = % HR^{max}

e.g.

180   - 204   x 100   = 88.2%

Where HR^{AT} from pg 41 = ☐

and HR^{max} from pg 41 = ☐

Convert % HR^{max} to VO_{2max} using the table below.

e.g.

88% HR^{max} = 75% VO_{2max}

Anaerobic threshold - % VO_{2max} = ☐

See 'Test results and analysis' table on page 167 for analysis.

Analysis Table

% Maximum Heartrate	%VO2^{max}
76	60
78	63
80	64
82	67
84	70
86	72
88	75
90	77
92	80
94	82
96	85
98	87
100	90

4.   Basic VO$_{2max}$ testing

At the point during exercise where you are consuming as much oxygen as you can get into your lungs, you have reached your VO$_{2max}$. This is the maximum (max) volume (vol) of oxygen (O$_2$) that you can can take in. VO$_{2max}$ measures the strength of your aerobic system your ability to take in oxygen.

This is a very basic running test to determine VO$_{2max}$. It's not a cycle test — for that you need a specifically calibrated cycle ergometer, and these are hard to find outside an exercise physiology lab. It is not the ideal test as it is not specific and not 100-percent accurate, but it doesn't require $100,000 worth of testing equipment and you don't have to be Einstein to calculate it.

Maximum Oxygen Uptake(MLO$_2$/Kg/Min)

MALES

Age/Rating	Excellent	Good	Average	Below Average	Poor
20-29	56 plus	51-55	44-50	38-43	34-37
30-39	52 plus	47-51	40-46	36-39	32-35
40-49	48 plus	43-47	36-42	32-35	28-31
50-59	45 plus	40-44	33-39	27-32	23-26
60-69	40 plus	35-39	28-34	24-27	20-23

FEMALES

Age/Rating	Excellent	Good	Average	Below Average	Poor
20-29	48 plus	45-47	38-44	33-37	29-32
30-39	45 plus	42-44	35-41	32-34	28-31
40-49	41 plus	38-40	31-37	28-30	24-27
50-59	38 plus	35-37	28-34	23-27	20-22
60-69	34 plus	31-33	24-30	21-23	17-20

Modified Margaria et al. run test formula

You need to record the distance you run and the time in which you complete it. The test must be done at the fastest pace you can hold for the full duration of the test (i.e. race pace). If you do this test:

1. Do not test over a distance less than 3000 m or more than 10,000 m.

2. Do a good warm-up and be very careful. Cyclists, rowers and other athletes who aren't used to running could get injured.

3. If you are at all worried about doing the test, consult a doctor before you do it. Doing the test if you are not prepared can be dangerous.

VO_{2max} (ml/kg/min) = [m + (30 x t)] / [5 (t + 1)]

where m = distance in metres; t = time in minutes.
(Seconds are expressed in decimal form; e.g. 30 seconds = 0.5 minutes.)
For example, 3000 m run in 12 minutes:

$$VO_{2max} = [3000 + (30 \times 12)] / [5 (12 + 1)]$$
$$= (3000 + 360) / (5 \times 13)$$
$$= 3360 / 65$$
$$= 51.7 \text{ ml/kg/min}$$

NOTE: You must be completely fresh to get an accurate result; even mild fatigue will reduce your score dramatically.

See appendix 1 for assessment of the result.
For example, 3000 m run in 12 minutes:
$$VO_{2max} = [3000 + (30 \times 12)] [5 (12 + 1)]$$
$$= (3000 + 360) / (5 \times 13)$$
$$= 3360 / 65$$
$$= 51.7 \text{ ml/kg/min}$$

Note: You must be completely fresh to get an accurate result; even mild fatigue will reduce your score dramatically.

See appendix 1 for assessment of the result. For more information, see *The Power to Perform.*

Appendix 4

Log book and training race analysis templates

The benefits of using a log book

The key to being a successful athlete is to train hard, train smart, and know what forms of training work for you.

Do you know how many weeks of speedwork you need to peak? Do you know what your optimal training, resting and racing heart rates are? Do you know what weekly programme format best suits you? Do you know when are the best times to race to peak effectively?

There are a huge number of questions that a properly constructed and used log book will answer. It will enable you to train smarter and race faster.

This log book acts as your personal coach. It asks you the questions your coach would ask to establish whether your training is working or not. It will teach you how to train far more effectively than ever before. Through analysis of your training you will be able to plan better and refine your training. With this you will be able to eliminate training errors and accentuate effective training. It will also provide a diary of previous build-ups to refer to, which you can use to set up your next training build-up. Ultimately you have a better understanding of your own body, your training and the requirements for racing to your full potential. All it requires is a little time spent planning and analysing your training each week. This is the future of training.

How to use your log book

This log book is set up with extensive training data collection techniques. It is designed so that it can be used by anyone from a world champion to a weekend warrior. You do not need to use all the facilities in the log book; use as many or as few as you like.

Daily log book usage

EACH MORNING BEFORE YOUR WORKOUT

Note down your resting pulse (taken in bed lying down upon waking) and your morning weight. These will help act as indicators to your training. Write these in pen on the far left of the page in the *Day/Date* section.

AFTER YOU HAVE COMPLETED YOUR WORKOUT

When you have completed your workout or workouts write the following information in the *Activity* section of your log book in pen to indicate its completion. There is space to write down specifics for up to three disciplines.

Fill out daily

- Time to complete the workout.
- Distance covered.
- Average speed, if you wish.
- Average training heart rate (if you have a pulse monitor). If you are doing speedwork, you may want to note down speedwork heart rates and average training heart rate separately.
- Under the *Specifics*, write in any important format points about your workout. This would mainly be used to note down intervals (distance, time, reps, sets) during speedwork.
- Under the *Specifics* fill out the total time for your workouts if you have completed more than one workout in the day. Also fill out the gym, stretching, and injury/illness questions by circling them if they apply. If they do not apply, ignore them.
- Next answer all the questions in the *Performance analysis* section by circling the word that most suits you. Be honest with yourself. The only person you are going to be fooling is you!
- In the *Comments* area in the *Performance analysis* section note down anything that you felt may not have been covered by the questions but that is of relevance.
- *Post-exercise weight* is also available in the *Performance analysis* section to aid in determining correct hydration techniques. If you weigh yourself immediately before and after you exercise, the weight difference is due to lack of adequate hydration. Drink 500 ml of fluid for every 500 g of weight lost. Remember that a 2-percent weight loss due to dehydration (1.4 kg in a 70 kg athlete) will seriously decrease performance and recovery.

NOTES: (a) Hills 1 2 3 and sprint 1 2 3: 1, 2 and 3 are measures of load. 1 means very, very hilly or maximum sprinting (<1 min); 2 is hilly or longer endurance sprints (1–4 min), and 3 means small hills or maximum steady-state pace speedwork (i.e. the fastest you can go without sprinting — 4 min+). (b) Sleep is in hours. (c) Post fatigue is when you feel good during your workout but feel very tired a few hours afterwards.

This may look like a lot to do but you will find that you can complete each day's entry in about two minutes — not much work for the amazing amount of specific practical information logged.

At the end of the week
Fill in the weekly summary in the same way as you have filled out the daily summary. You will find that because of the set-up of the log book it is easy to identify training errors and strengths. The log book is set up so that you are looking for patterns in the circling of information rather than having to read the whole week's notes. It will take you about five minutes to fill out.

WEEKLY SUMMARY

- Note down the week number (number of weeks into your build-up).
- Work out averages for weight, resting pulse, sleep, and training time/distance. See Appendix 9D if you are not sure how to calculate this.
- Estimate the percentage increase or decrease in training volume using total training time/distance and last week's total. Note this down as '% increase/decrease'. See Appendix 9E if you are not sure how to calculate this. This is useful for determining whether you are increasing your training volumes too quickly. Fill out the other questions by circling the word that is most appropriate.

TRAINING NOTES
Make any other relevant notes on your training under *Training notes*.

Racing
Answer each of the questions in the *Racing* pages of the log book (fig. A4.1). Rate your personal performance on a scale of one to five. One means that you were very happy with your performance and five means that you were very unhappy with your performance.

Calculate percentage field. This is useful for determining your performance on different courses against different numbers of competitors. It does help to standardise your results if it is difficult to check this any other way. Also available separately as "The Performance Log."

DAY	ACTIVITY			PERFORMANCE ANALYSIS
MON **DATE** **H.R.** **WGHT**	SPORT TIME: DIST: AV SPEED: AV H.R. SPECIFICS: TOTAL TIME: _____	SPORT TIME: DIST: AV SPEED: AV H.R. SPECIFICS: Stretching / Injury / Illness	SPORT TIME: DIST: AV SPEED: AV H.R. SPECIFICS:	FELT: Excellent/Good/Average/Tired/V.Tired STRESS: Mellow/Moderate/High/VHigh BENEFIT: Excellent/Good/Average/Poor/☺☹ SLEEP: 11,10,9,8,7,6,5,4,3 Good/Average/Broken NUTRITION: Good/Average/Poor/Binge Day AIM: Base – Long/Hills 1 2 3/Easy/Technique Speed – Race/Time Trial/Intervals/Sprint 1 2 3 INTENSITY: >100%,100%,90%,80%,70%,60%,50% WEATHER: Calm/Moderate/Windy/Wet/Cold/Hot WATER: Calm/Moderate/Rough COMMENTS:
	GYM:Weights –	Strength/Circuit	Aerobics/Flex	Post Exercise Weight:
TUES **DATE** **H.R.** **WGHT**	SPORT TIME: DIST: AV SPEED: AV H.R. SPECIFICS: TOTAL TIME: _____	SPORT TIME: DIST: AV SPEED: AV H.R. SPECIFICS: Stretching / Injury / Illness	SPORT TIME: DIST: AV SPEED: AV H.R. SPECIFICS:	FELT: Excellent/Good/Average/Tired/V.Tired STRESS: Mellow/Moderate/High/VHigh BENEFIT: Excellent/Good/Average/Poor/☺☹ SLEEP: 11,10,9,8,7,6,5,4,3 Good/Average/Broken NUTRITION: Good/Average/Poor/Binge Day AIM: Base – Long/Hills 1 2 3/Easy/Technique Speed – Race/Time Trial/Intervals/Sprint 1 2 INTENSITY: >100%,100%,90%,80%,70%,60%,50% WEATHER: Calm/Moderate/Windy/Wet/Cold/Hot WATER: Calm/Moderate/Rough COMMENTS:
	GYM:Weights –	Strength/Circuit	Aerobics/Flex	Post Exercise Weight:
WED **DATE** **H.R.** **WGHT**	SPORT TIME: DIST: AV SPEED: AV H.R. SPECIFICS: TOTAL TIME: _____	SPORT TIME: DIST: AV SPEED: AV H.R. SPECIFICS: Stretching / Injury / Illness	SPORT TIME: DIST: AV SPEED: AV H.R. SPECIFICS:	FELT: Excellent/Good/Average/Tired/V.Tired STRESS: Mellow/Moderate/High/VHigh BENEFIT: Excellent/Good/Average/Poor/☺☹ SLEEP: 11,10,9,8,7,6,5,4,3 Good/Average/Broken NUTRITION: Good/Average/Poor/Binge Day AIM: Base – Long/Hills 1 2 3/Easy/Technique Speed – Race/Time Trial/Intervals/Sprint 1 2 3 INTENSITY: >100%,100%,90%,80%,70%,60%,50% WEATHER: Calm/Moderate/Windy/Wet/Cold/Hot WATER: Calm/Moderate/Rough COMMENTS:
	GYM:Weights –	Strength/Circuit	Aerobics/Flex	Post Exercise Weight:
THUR **DATE** **H.R.** **WGHT**	SPORT TIME: DIST: AV SPEED: AV H.R. SPECIFICS: TOTAL TIME: _____	SPORT TIME: DIST: AV SPEED: AV H.R. SPECIFICS: Stretching / Injury / Illness	SPORT TIME: DIST: AV SPEED: AV H.R. SPECIFICS:	FELT: Excellent/Good/Average/Tired/V.Tired STRESS: Mellow/Moderate/High/VHigh BENEFIT: Excellent/Good/Average/Poor/☺☹ SLEEP: 11,10,9,8,7,6,5,4,3 Good/Average/Broken NUTRITION: Good/Average/Poor/Binge Day AIM: Base – Long/Hills 1 2 3/Easy/Technique Speed – Race/Time Trial/Intervals/Sprint 1 2 3 INTENSITY: >100%,100%,90%,80%,70%,60%,50% WEATHER: Calm/Moderate/Windy/Wet/Cold/Hot WATER: Calm/Moderate/Rough COMMENTS:
	GYM:Weights –	Strength/Circuit	Aerobics/Flex	Post Exercise Weight:

ACTIVITY			PERFORMANCE ANALYSIS	DAY

SPORT	SPORT	SPORT	FELT: Excellent/Good/Average/Tired/V.Tired	
			STRESS: Mellow/Moderate/High/VHigh	**FRI**
TIME:	TIME:	TIME:	BENEFIT: Excellent/Good/Average/Poor/☺☹	
DIST:	DIST:	DIST:	SLEEP: 11,10,9,8,7,6,5,4,3 Good/Average/Broken	
			NUTRITION: Good/Average/Poor/Binge Day	**DATE**
AV SPEED:	AV SPEED:	AV SPEED:	AIM: Base – Long/Hills 1 2 3/Easy/Technique	
			Speed – Race/Time Trial/Intervals/Sprint 1 2 3	**H.R.**
AV H.R.	AV H.R.	AV H.R.	INTENSITY: >100%,100%,90%,80%,70%,60%,50%	
SPECIFICS:	SPECIFICS:	SPECIFICS:	WEATHER: Calm/Moderate/Windy/Wet/Cold/Hot	**WGHT**
			WATER: Calm/Moderate/Rough	
			COMMENTS:	
TOTAL TIME: _____ Stretching / Injury / Illness				
GYM: Weights – Strength/Circuit Aerobics/Flex			Post Exercise Weight:	

SPORT	SPORT	SPORT	FELT: Excellent/Good/Average/Tired/V.Tired	
			STRESS: Mellow/Moderate/High/VHigh	**SAT**
TIME:	TIME:	TIME:	BENEFIT: Excellent/Good/Average/Poor/☺☹	
DIST:	DIST:	DIST:	SLEEP: 11,10,9,8,7,6,5,4,3 Good/Average/Broken	
			NUTRITION: Good/Average/Poor/Binge Day	**DATE**
AV SPEED:	AV SPEED:	AV SPEED:	AIM: Base – Long/Hills 1 2 3/Easy/Technique	
			Speed – Race/Time Trial/Intervals/Sprint 1 2 3	**H.R.**
AV H.R.	AV H.R.	AV H.R.	INTENSITY: >100%,100%,90%,80%,70%,60%,50%	
SPECIFICS:	SPECIFICS:	SPECIFICS:	WEATHER: Calm/Moderate/Windy/Wet/Cold/Hot	**WGHT**
			WATER: Calm/Moderate/Rough	
			COMMENTS:	
TOTAL TIME: _____ Stretching / Injury / Illness				
GYM: Weights – Strength/Circuit Aerobics/Flex			Post Exercise Weight:	

SPORT	SPORT	SPORT	FELT: Excellent/Good/Average/Tired/V.Tired	
			STRESS: Mellow/Moderate/High/VHigh	**SUN**
TIME:	TIME:	TIME:	BENEFIT: Excellent/Good/Average/Poor/☺☹	
DIST:	DIST:	DIST:	SLEEP: 11,10,9,8,7,6,5,4,3 Good/Average/Broken	
			NUTRITION: Good/Average/Poor/Binge Day	**DATE**
AV SPEED:	AV SPEED:	AV SPEED:	AIM: Base – Long/Hills 1 2 3/Easy/Technique	
			Speed – Race/Time Trial/Intervals/Sprint 1 2 3	**H.R.**
AV H.R.	AV H.R.	AV H.R.	INTENSITY: >100%,100%,90%,80%,70%,60%,50%	
SPECIFICS:	SPECIFICS:	SPECIFICS:	WEATHER: Calm/Moderate/Windy/Wet/Cold/Hot	**WGHT**
			WATER: Calm/Moderate/Rough	
			COMMENTS:	
TOTAL TIME: _____ Stretching / Injury / Illness				
GYM: Weights – Strength/Circuit Aerobics/Flex			Post Exercise Weight:	

WEEKLY SUMMARY

WEEK NO: _____
WEIGHT (AV): _____
REST PULSE (AV): _____
SLEEP (AV): _____
TRAINING TIME/DIST (AV): _____
TOTAL TRAINING TIME/DIST: _____
LAST WEEKS TOTAL: _____
% INCREASE/DECREASE: _____
PHYSICAL CONDITION: Excellent/Good/Average/Groan!
STRESS: Mellow/Moderate/High
EFFECTIVENESS: Excellent/Good/Average/☺☹
NUTRITION: Good/Moderate/Poor

TRAINING NOTES

_____
_____
_____
_____
_____
_____
_____
_____
_____
_____
_____
_____

RACE: _____   PERFORMANCE: 1 2 3 4 5
PLACE: _____ % FIELD _____ TOTAL FIELD _____
DISTS: 1 _____ 2 _____ 3 _____   4 _____
          1 _____ TRAN _____ 2 _____   TRAN _____
          3 _____ TRAN _____ 4 _____   TOTAL _____
AV SPEED: COURSE: hilly 1 2 3 / flat
WEATHER: hot / cold / wet / windy / moderate / calm
WATER: calm / moderate / rough   AV H.R. _____
EQUIPMENT SET-UP: _____

RACE: _____   PERFORMANCE: 1 2 3 4 5
PLACE: _____ % FIELD _____ TOTAL FIELD _____
DISTS: 1 _____ 2 _____ 3 _____   4 _____
          1 _____ TRAN _____ 2 _____   TRAN _____
          3 _____ TRAN _____ 4 _____   TOTAL _____
AV SPEED: COURSE: hilly 1 2 3 / flat
WEATHER: hot / cold / wet / windy / moderate / calm
WATER: calm / moderate / rough   AV H.R. _____
EQUIPMENT SET-UP: _____

RACE: _____   PERFORMANCE: 1 2 3 4 5
PLACE: _____ % FIELD _____ TOTAL FIELD _____
DISTS: 1 _____ 2 _____ 3 _____   4 _____
          1 _____ TRAN _____ 2 _____   TRAN _____
          3 _____ TRAN _____ 4 _____   TOTAL _____
AV SPEED: COURSE: hilly 1 2 3 / flat
WEATHER: hot / cold / wet / windy / moderate / calm
WATER: calm / moderate / rough   AV H.R. _____
EQUIPMENT SET-UP: _____

RACE: _____   PERFORMANCE: 1 2 3 4 5
PLACE: _____ % FIELD _____ TOTAL FIELD _____
DISTS: 1 _____ 2 _____ 3 _____   4 _____
          1 _____ TRAN _____ 2 _____   TRAN _____
          3 _____ TRAN _____ 4 _____   TOTAL _____
AV SPEED: COURSE: hilly 1 2 3 / flat
WEATHER: hot / cold / wet / windy / moderate / calm
WATER: calm / moderate / rough   AV H.R. _____
EQUIPMENT SET-UP: _____

Fig A4.1 Racing analysis